Stroke Prevention
in Clinical Practice

W0080680

Stroke Prevention in Clinical Practice

Daryll M. Baker

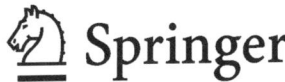 Springer

Daryll M. Baker, PhD, FRCS
Consultant Vascular Surgeon
Royal Free Hospital
London, UK

British Library Cataloguing in Publication Data
Baker, Daryll M.
Stroke prevention in clinical practice 1. Cerebrovascular disease –
Prevention 2. Cerebrovascular disease – Diagnosis 3. Cerebrovascular
disease – Treatment 4. Transient ischemic attack – Diagnosis
I. Title
616.8'105

Library of Congress Control Number: 2007926595

ISBN 978-1-85233-964-7   e-ISBN 978-1-84628-728-2

Printed on acid-free paper

9 8 7 6 5 4 3 2 1

Springer Science+Business Media
springer.com

Preface

Stroke is the third most common cause of death in the world. Furthermore, for those who survive, stroke is the most common cause of severe disability, such that after a year, 25% are still dependent on someone else for everyday activities, and within 5 years, a third of these will have suffered a second stroke.

Clearly, every effort to reduce the incidence and severity of stroke needs to be taken.

This handbook considers the different ways of reducing the risk of ischaemic stroke. A summary of the significance of each risk factor is followed by an outline on how to make the diagnosis both on the basis of clinical features and with investigations. How to modify the risk factor is then considered along with the associated risks of intervention and evidence for the recommendation. Relevant references are given if more detailed information is required.

Contents

Part I
Introduction

Chapter 1
The Significance of Stroke

> Stroke is a common disease with a high morbidity and mortality. All efforts to reduce its occurrence need to be undertaken.

DEFINITION

Stroke is a clinical syndrome associated with the sudden loss of focal brain function for more than 24 hours. It is caused by an interruption in the blood supply to the affected brain area (ischemic stroke) or by a spontaneous hemorrhage into or over the brain (a hemorrhagic stroke).

A transient ischemic attack (TIA) is a syndrome associated with the sudden loss of focal brain or monocular function lasting less than 24 hours, and usually only a few minutes.

Amaurosis fugax is a TIA of the eye and is sudden transient monocular blindness.

INCIDENCE

The incidence of first stroke is 200 per 100,000 per year (0.2% of the population). The incidence of cerebral TIA is 50 per 100,000 per year. The incidence of stroke is influenced by the following:

1. Age: the incidence rises rapidly with increased age, with one quarter occurring before the age of 65 years and one half before the age of 75 years.
2. Race: the incidence of all strokes is higher in blacks. This may be due to a higher prevalence of risk factors such as hypertension, diabetes, obesity and sickle cell trait in blacks than in whites.
3. Geographical variations: there is a higher incidence of stroke in Eastern Europe and China than in France.

Sex is not a factor, as stroke has an equal distribution.

PREVALENCE

The prevalence depends on the incidence and survival. The prevalence of stroke is 5 to 12 per 1000 population, but is higher with increased age, and in males and black populations.

MORBIDITY

Disability from Stroke

Stroke is the most important cause of severe disability in England and Wales.

With good rehabilitation, neurological function often begins to improve within a few days of the stroke and continues to improve, especially within the first 3 months. After this period, improvement is at a slower rate, and at 1 to 2 years only minimal improvement is achieved.

A year after a stroke, 25% of patients are dependent on someone else for everyday activities such as dressing, washing, and mobilizing, but 50% do live independently. On an individual basis this depends not only on the magnitude of the stroke and degree of recovery, but also on the premorbid disabilities and social support available.

Risk of Recurrent Stroke

Despite undertaking all stroke preventative measures the risk of a recurrent stroke remains. This is around 3% in the first month, and 15% within the first year, but falls to 5% per year thereafter, so that at 5 years 30% will have suffered a second stroke.

Risk of Cardiovascular Disease

After a stroke, 5% to 10% of patients suffer a myocardial infarct each year.

MORTALITY

Stroke is the third commonest cause of death throughout the world, after coronary heart disease and all cancers. There are five million deaths a year from stroke, 75% of which occur in the developing world.

Twenty-five percent of all stroke patients are dead within a year of their first stroke, which accounts for 12% of deaths, an incidence of 60 per 100,000 population per year in England and Wales.

ETIOLOGY AND TYPES OF ISCHEMIC STROKE

Stroke is caused by occlusion of a feeder end artery. The occlusion is the result of either an embolus from elsewhere or an in-situ occlusion.

Common causes of a TIA or ischemic stroke are as follows:

1. Large artery atherosclerotic thromboembolism—50%
     Extra-cranial (aorta, carotid, vertebral arteries)—45%
     Intracranial vessels—5%
2. Cardiac thromboembolism—20%
3. Lacunar syndromes (small vessel occlusion)—25%
4. Nonatheromatous arterial disease (dissection, arteritis)—5%
5. Hematological disorders—<5%

Chapter 2

Identifying Patients at Risk of Ischemic Stroke

> People at a high risk of stroke need to be identified and treated.

With an incidence of first stroke at 200 per 100,000 per year, most people are at some risk of stroke, but certain groups can be identified who are at a much higher risk than others.

There are several ischemic stroke risk factors (Fig. 2.1), some of which are not amenable to prevention, but still provide a strong indication of patients at risk. Other factors are risks as they provide a source of cerebral emboli and other factors are of importance as they are associated with progression of atherosclerosis or in a few cases thrombosis.

The patients at highest risk of stroke should be targeted first with regard to stroke prevention interventions. They include those with previous cerebrovascular events (stroke or transient ischemic attacks) and other groups, including those with atrial fibrillation, hypertension and diabetes.

PATIENTS WITH PREVIOUS CEREBROVASCULAR EVENTS

Of the risk factors outlined in Fig. 2.1, the most significant is the history of a previous cerebrovascular event. Although this event cannot be prevented, the associated high risk of a further event means these patients need to be clearly identified, and any associated risk factors treated.

Patients with Previous Stroke

The risk of recurrent stroke after the first cerebral infarction is 2% at 7 days, 4% at 30 days, 12% at 1 year, and 29% at 5 years. This

I. Non-modifiable stroke risk factors

1. Age
2. Family history of cerebrovascular events
3. Ethnicity
4. Geographical location
5. Previous cerebrovascular events

II. Cerebrovascular embolic risk factors

1. Cardio-embolic risk factors
   a. Atrial fibrillation
   b. Valvular diseases
3. Infective endocarditis
   c. Myocardial infarct
   d. Other mural disorders such as chronic cardiac failure, patent foramen ovale, cardiac tumours
2. Major artery embolic risk factors
   a. Carotid artery stenosis
   b. Carotid artery dissection
   c. Vertebrobasilar artery stenosis
   d. Aortic arch atheroma

III. Atherosclerotic cerebrovascular risk factors

1. Stroke risk factors which can be influenced
   1. Hypertension
   2. Diabetes,
   3. Hyperlipidaemia
   4. hyper-homocystineaemia
2. Risk factors that can be treated by life style changes
   1. Obesity
   2. Physical inactivity
   3. Cigarette smoking
   4. Others oral contraceptive medications,
3. Patients with other cardiovascular disease Including peripheral vascular disease and ischaemic heart disease

IV. Hypercoagulabile risk factors

Thrombophilia
Sickle cell

FIGURE 2.1. Ischaemic stroke risk factors.

risk is higher if the stroke is associated with any of the following factors:

1. Advancing age
2. If the stroke is hemorrhagic

3. There is a history of previous transient ischemic attack (TIA)
4. Dementia develops after the stroke
5. Other cerebrovascular risk factors, such as hypertension, diabetes, cigarette smoking, and atrial fibrillation, are present

Transient Ischemic Attacks

Transient ischemic attacks have the same demographic distribution, long-term prognosis, and associated vascular risk factors as stroke, and therefore the need to ensure that stroke preventative measures are taken is the same.

The distinction between TIA and stroke is important because of the following factors:

1. TIAs are reported less often than a stroke and therefore require a more careful history.
2. The differential diagnoses for stroke and TIA differ.
3. A diagnosis of TIA is often less accurate than that of stroke, as it relies on only the history.

SIGNIFICANCE OF A TRANSIENT ISCHEMIC ATTACK

Transient ischemic attack patients have a 5% risk of stroke in the first month, 12% in 12 months, and 30% over 5 years, which is seven times the matched population risk and the same risk as a full stroke. They have an increased risk of a cardiac event of around 3% per year.

In combination, the risk of a serious vascular event (stroke, myocardial infarct, or death due to vascular cause) following a TIA is 10% per year. This risk is greater in those with any of the following:

1. Cerebral TIAs rather than amaurosis fugax
2. Repeated TIAs over a short period
3. Increased age
4. Carotid stenosis
5. Peripheral vascular disease

DIAGNOSING A TRANSIENT ISCHEMIC ATTACK

The diagnosis requires a careful history, as presentation usually occurs more than 24 hours after onset, and the signs have resolved.

The distinguishing symptomatic features of a TIA include the following:

1. Focal rather than nonfocal neurology (Fig. 2.2). The commonest symptom is unilateral weakness, heaviness, or clumsiness, which occurs in half the patients. Unilateral sensory symptoms occur in a third of patients, and slurred speech in one quarter. Transient monocular blindness is reported in a fifth of patients.
2. A neurological deficit rather than a gain of function, for example, weakness, numbness, blindness as opposed to jerking, paresthesia, flashing visual lights
3. Sudden onset
4. No clinical signs; it has completely resolved.

Once the diagnosis of a TIA has been made, assessing the anatomical distribution of the neurological deficit gives an indication of the brain territory involved. This is usually considered as an anterior (carotid) or posterior (vertebrobasilar) TIA. This is helpful in assessing the potential need for a carotid endarterectomy; however, there is much variability, as there are not only anatomical variants (such as one particular carotid giving rise to the anterior, middle, and posterior cerebral arteries in 15% of cases), but also interclinician variability in determining which collection of symptoms is attributable to a carotid or vertebral circulation disturbance.

Focal neurological symptoms

a. Anterior (Carotid) distribution (80%)
   Weakness or clumsiness of one side of the body
   Dysphasia (difficulty understanding or expressing the spoken word)
   Dyslexia (difficulty reading) Dysgraphia (difficulty writing)
   Transient monocular blindness (loss of vision in one eye in whole or in part)
b. Posterior (Vertebrobasilar) distribution (20%) Motor / sensory deficits affecting any extremity including crossed face and limbs, bilaterally
   Bilateral visual loss

Non focal neurological symptoms

Generalised weakness and or sensory disturbances
Light headedness / faintness
"Blackouts" with altered loss of consciousness
Incontinence of urine or faeces
Confusion

FIGURE 2.2. Symptoms of a cerebrovascular event.

TRANSIENT ISCHEMIC ATTACK DIFFERENTIAL DIAGNOSIS

Clinical symptoms that suggest a differential diagnoses need to be borne in mind:

Migraine

Distinguishing features include:

1. Neurological symptoms:
   a. Tend to be positive, such as tingling and visual aura
   b. May spread to adjacent areas over minutes rather than occurring simultaneously and immediately
2. Other symptoms
   a. Headache, which is unilateral pulsatile
   b. Nausea often following neurology events
   c. A past or family history of migraine
   d. Symptoms tend to occur in a young age group with no vascular risk factors

Partial Epileptic Seizures

Distinguishing features include:

1. Neurological symptoms
   a. Positive symptoms, e.g., limb jerking
   b. Can arise over few moments, not abruptly
   c. Spread to adjacent areas over a few seconds
   d. May progress to full generalized tonic-clonic convulsion or loss of consciousness
2. Other symptoms
   a. There may be a prodrome, such as epigastric discomfort before partial seizure symptoms develop

Transient Global Amnesia

Distinguishing features include

1. Neurological symptoms
   a. An abrupt loss of short-term memory, but with no reduced level of consciousness, loss of personal identity, or ability to recognize familiar objects or perform repetitive tasks.
   b. Resolves within 24 hours
   c. No focal neurological features
2. Other symptoms
   a. Often repetitive questioning
   b. Rarely recurs

Middle Ear Disorders

Middle ear disorders include acute labyrinthitis, benign recurrent vertigo, and benign paroxysmal positional vertigo. Distinguishing features include:

1. Neurological symptoms
   a. Vertigo with ataxia associated with no other neurological features
   b. Can last longer than 24 hours
2. Other symptoms include nausea

Drop Attacks

Distinguishing features include:

1. Neurological symptoms
   a. No focal neurological features
   b. No loss of consciousness
   c. Recovery is immediate
2. Other features
   a. Occurs mainly in middle-aged women in whom the legs give way and the patient falls to the ground
   b. Only occurs when upright

Syncope

Distinguishing features include:

1. No focal neurological features
2. Usually a clear precipitating event

AMAUROSIS FUGAX DIFFERENTIAL DIAGNOSIS

If there is any question about the diagnosis and funduscopy is not helpful, an ophthalmic opinion should be sought.

Retinal Migraine

Distinguishing features include:

1. Eye symptoms:
   a. Monocular visual impairment gradually worsens but is rarely complete
   b. Associated with positive visual symptoms such as flashing lights
2. Other features
   a. Pulsatile headache
   b. Orbital pain

Central Retinal Vein Thrombosis
Can be associated with transient monocular blindness but the differential diagnosis is made by funduscopy.

Retinal Hemorrhages
If these hemorrhages are the cause of sudden monocular loss of vision, they are rarely transient.

Other Causes of Monocular Blindness
Other causes are usually not transient and involve specific ocular pathology including glaucoma, anterior ischemic optic neuropathy due to arteritis, and anterior or posterior chamber hemorrhages.

INVESTIGATIONS TO MAKE THE DIAGNOSIS OF TRANSIENT ISCHEMIC ATTACK
The diagnosis of TIA is made on the history, with the clinical examination and investigations being normal and therefore not usually necessary.

Computed tomography (CT) brain imaging is undertaken to detect underlying structural intracranial lesions, such as arteriovenous malformations, meningiomas, subdural hematomas (detects lesion in 1% of suspected TIAs), and not to detect infarct lesions or to exclude primary intracerebral bleeds.

HOW WELL IS TRANSIENT ISCHEMIC ATTACK DIAGNOSED?
Primary care physicians' clinical diagnosis of a TIA has been felt to be inaccurate by neurologists in up to 60% of cases; however, considerable intraneurologist variability in making the diagnosis has also been found. This is because the diagnosis is reliant on the history only and there are no clear features.

OTHER PATIENTS AT RISK OF A CEREBROVASCULAR EVENT
All interventions carry risks, and therefore as part of the risk–benefit assessment it is common to consider stroke prevention to be either primary or secondary. Primary prevention is recommended in patients who have yet to suffer a cerebrovascular event, and secondary prevention is recommended for those patients who have suffered a stroke. However, some patients are at high risk of stroke even if they have yet to suffer a full stroke, and aggressive

intervention is recommended. Such groups are considered in later chapters and include those with

1. Atrial fibrillation
2. Hypertension
3. Diabetes
4. Smoking
5. Other cardiovascular diseases

Chapter 3
Investigating Patients at Risk of Stroke

Patients at highest risk of stroke are those who have already suffered a cerebrovascular event, those in atrial fibrillation, and those with hypertension or diabetes.

Investigations are aimed at identifying these groups of patients and identifying other modifiable cerebrovascular risk factors.

A battery of primary investigations needs to be considered on all patients at risk of stroke, and then secondary investigations selected according to the individual case.

PRIMARY INVESTIGATIONS

1. Vascular Imaging
   a. Carotid duplex ultrasound scanning: a duplex ultrasound machine produces both B-mode images, which give an indication of the anatomical shape of the vessel and its contained stenosis, and Doppler mode images, which give an impression of disturbances in flow. Together they identify:
      i. Carotid artery stenoses and dissections
      ii. Vertebral artery origin stenoses and the direction of vertebral flow.
2. Cardiac imaging
   a. Transthoracic cardiac echo to identify a cardiac source of cerebral emboli
   b. Chest x-ray to identify cardiac enlargement in hypertension and valvular disease
   c. Electrocardiogram (ECG), possibly a 24-hour ECG to exclude runs of atrial fibrillation
3. Laboratory blood tests
   a. Full blood count to exclude anemia, polycythemia, and thrombocytopenia
   b. Blood glucose to identify diabetes
   c. Serum lipid profile.
   d. Erythrocyte sedimentation rate as a screen for a vasculitis
   e. Serum biochemistry

SECONDARY INVESTIGATIONS

1. Brain imaging: computed tomography (CT) and magnetic resonance imaging (MRI) are indicated if the diagnosis of a previous cerebrovascular event is in doubt, if there is a question as to whether the event was hemorrhagic rather than ischemic in nature, and if an arterial dissection is suspected.
2. Vascular imaging
   a. Transcranial duplex ultrasound to demonstrate cerebral artery blockage especially in sickle cell patients
   b. Magnetic resonance angiography
   c. Digital subtraction angiography
3. Cardiac assessment
   a. Transesophageal cardiac echo is considered if an embolic source is suspected in the venous system, left atrium, or aortic arch
   b. 24-hour ambulatory blood pressure monitoring
4. Laboratory blood test
   a. Coagulation defects
      i. Sickle cell screen
      ii. Coagulation profile and thrombophilia screen
      iii. plasma electrophoresis and viscosity studies in myeloma
   b. Autoantibody screen for a suspected vasculitis, collagen vascular disease
   c. Syphilis and HIV serology
   d. Fasting plasma homocysteine
   e. Fasting blood glucose, glycosylated hemoglobin (HbA_{1C}).
   f. Blood cultures in suspected infective endocarditis
5. Urine analysis

This is not a complete list and other tests need to be added if a more elusive diagnosis is suspected.

Part II
Reducing the Risk of Stroke
by Reducing Embolic Events

Chapter 4
Antiplatelet Therapy

Recommendations

1. All patients who have had an ischaemic cerebrovascular event should be on antiplatelet therapy.
2. First-line treatment is low-dose aspirin (75 to 150 mg/ day).
3. If no other vascular beds are involved dipyridamole SR (200mg b.i.d.) should be taken as well.
4. If there are symptoms on therapy and/or intolerance to aspirin, clopidogrel (75 mg/day) should be used.
5. There is little evidence to support the use of aspirin and clopidogrel in combination.

Platelets aggregate at the site of endothelial damage and plug the gaps between activated fibrin strands to stop bleeding. Platelets also aggregate on exposure to subendothelial collagen or the contents of ruptured atheromatous plaques, leading to the occlusion of the vessel or the showering of emboli downstream, both of which can result in a stroke if the cerebral vessels are involved.

SIGNIFICANCE
Antiplatelet therapy reduces platelet aggregation and therefore the likelihood of further stroke.

Evidence: The Antiplatelet Trialist Collaboration meta-analysis demonstrated that antiplatelet therapy reduces the risk of nonfatal stroke by 25% in patients with a previous cerebrovascular event.

TREATMENT

Who Should Be Treated?

Primary Prevention
Patients who have not suffered a cerebrovascular event but have manifestations of atherosclerotic disease in other vascular beds such as ischemic heart disease or peripheral vascular disease will benefit from taking antiplatelet medications to reduce the risk of an event not only in these beds but also in the cerebrovascular system. In those with significant cardiovascular risk factors, such as diabetes or hypertension, antiplatelet therapy should also be considered.

Secondary Prevention
All patients who have had an ischemic cerebrovascular event should be on antiplatelet therapy.

Which Drug Should Be Used?
There are three classes of antiplatelet drugs available: aspirin, dipyridamole, and clopidogrel.

Aspirin
Indication. First-line antiplatelet therapy.

Dose. Low dose (75-150 mg) per day.

Mode of Action. Aspirin is a cyclooxygenase enzyme inhibitor that acetylates the cyclooxygenase enzyme resulting in a decrease in prostacyclin and thromboxane synthesis within the platelet. It does not inhibit the resynthesis of cyclooxygenase in the vascular endothelium, so endothelium-derived prostacyclin is available to inhibit platelet adhesion.

Rationale. Aspirin reduces the likelihood of stroke, which is probably independent of dose.

Evidence: A meta-analysis by the Antiplatelet Trialist Collaboration found that for a patient with a previous cerebrovascular event who takes aspirin, the absolute risk reduction of a serious vascular event (nonfatal myocardial infarction, nonfatal stroke, or vascular death) is 1% per year (reduction from an average of 7% to 6% per year). The number needed to treat to prevent one stroke is about 100. The analysis also demonstrated that lower doses (75–100 mg/day) were as effective as higher doses

Side Effects

1. Gastrointestinal bleed: Hematemesis attributable to aspirin occurs in 0.5 per 1000 person years of aspirin exposure, that is, a relative excess risk of 70%. It is probable that higher doses of aspirin are associated with a higher risk of gastrointestinal bleed compared with medium doses, but this is not the case for low doses when compared with medium doses. The risk is probably independent of preparation modification. It occurs predominantly from bleeds in the gastric mucosa, and the incidence is higher in patients concurrently using nonsteroidal antiinflammatory drugs (NSAIDs) and those taking clopidogrel concurrently.
2. Abdominal discomfort: Up to 30% of patients taking aspirin experience some upper gastrointestinal discomfort, such as nausea, heartburn, and epigastric pain, which could be related to gastric mucosal irritation, but in controlled trials 20% of those taking a placebo also reported similar symptoms. These symptoms may be dose related.
3. Intracranial hemorrhage is uncommon, with an incidence of 1 per 1000 aspirin takers over 3 years.
4. Bronchospasm can occur, and therefore aspirin should be used with caution in asthmatics
5. About 5% of patients cannot tolerate aspirin or are allergic to it.

Dipyridamole
Indications

1. In combination with aspirin in patients who have suffered a cerebrovascular event, especially if there is no associated ischemic heart disease
2. In patients whom have a high risk of bleeding

Dose. Modified release, 200 mg BD.

Mode of Action. Probably by increasing circulating adenosine diphosphate (ADP) availability.

Evidence:

1. *Dipyridamole in combination with low-dose aspirin significantly reduces the incidence of a further cerebrovascular event (relative risk [RR] 37%) compared with an RR of 16% if used alone and an RR of 18% for aspirin alone as compared with no antiplatelet treatment.*
2. *Subsequent meta-analysis suggested that dipyridamole does not appear to reduce the risk of events in other vascular beds (e.g., ischemic heart disease, or peripheral vascular disease)*

Side Effects

1. Gastrointestinal upset, such as nausea and diarrhea is the cause of discontinuing treatment in 7%
2. Throbbing headache and dizziness

Clopidogrel
Indications

1. Patients intolerant to aspirin will gain some stroke protection by taking clopidogrel.
2. In patients who have significant disease in several vascular beds as well as having suffered as cerebrovascular event, including ischemic heart disease and peripheral vascular disease, clopidogrel can be taken to reduce the rate of progression of atherosclerosis symptoms in these beds.

Dose. 75 mg a day.

Mode of Action. Selectively inhibits ADP-induced platelet aggregation.

Evidence: Clopidogrel alone is no better than aspirin at reducing the incidence of secondary cerebrovascular events, although it does offer greater protection when considering a combination of secondary atherosclerotic events (e.g., a composite of ischemic stroke, myocardial infarction, vascular death, and rehospitalization for acute ischemia event) (CAPRIE [Clopidogrel vs. Aspirin in Patients at Risk of Ischemic Events] trial)
Clopidogrel in combination with aspirin adds no benefit to stroke prevention (MATCH [Management of A Therothrombosis with clopidogrel in High-risk Pateints with recent TIA or is Chemic Stroke] trial) and is associated with higher intracerebral bleeds, although clopidogrel in combination with aspirin does appear to offer even greater protection against cardiac events.

Side Effects (Alone and in Combination with Aspirin)

1. Gastrointestinal hemorrhage: clopidogrel has a lower incidence of gastrointestinal hemorrhage than aspirin (0.5% vs. 0.9%)
2. Abdominal discomfort with associated nausea and vomiting and altered bowel habit
3. Rash (1%)
4. Headache, dizziness and vertigo

Other Antiplatelet Agents
1. Ticlopidine, which is structurally similar to clopidogrel, reduces stroke, myocardial infarction, and vascular deaths probably to a greater extent than aspirin, but is associated with an unacceptably high incidence of neutropenia.

2. Other agents such as the Glycoprotein IIB/IIa receptor antagonists are not effective in secondary stroke prevention.
3. Warfarin: There is no place for warfarin use as secondary prevention against a recurrent cerebrovascular event in patients without atrial fibrillation. Although warfarin could be used in patients who are unable to take aspirin, the use of other antiplatelet drugs is recommended.

Bibliography

Antithrombotic Trialists' Collaboration Collaborative meta-analysis of randomised trials of antiplatelet therapy for prevention of death, myocardial infarction, and stroke in high risk patients. BMJ 2002;324(7329):71–86.

De Schryver EL, Algra A, van Gijn J. Dipyridamole for preventing stroke and other vascular events in patients with vascular disease. Cochrane Database Syst Rev 2003;(1):CD001820.

Diener HC, Bogousslavsky J, Brass LM, et al., MATCH investigators. Aspirin and clopidogrel compared with clopidogrel alone after recent ischaemic stroke or transient ischaemic attack in high-risk patients (MATCH): randomised, double-blind, placebo-controlled trial. Lancet 2004;364(9431):331–337.

Ringleb PA, Bhatt DL, Hirsch AT, Topol EJ, Hacke W, for the CAPRIE investigators. Benefit of clopidogrel over aspirin is amplified in patients with a history of ischemic events. Stroke 2004;35:528.

Sandercock P, Mielke O, Liu M, Counsell C. Anticoagulants for preventing recurrence following presumed non-cardioembolic ischaemic stroke or transient ischaemic attack. Cochrane Database Syst Rev 2002;(4):CD000248.

Chapter 5
Reducing Cardioembolic Events

Recommendations

The heart is an important source of ischemic stroke emboli. It therefore needs to be fully assessed following any cerebrovascular event.

Although cardiac emboli can be distributed throughout the body, 80% of symptomatic cardiac emboli involve the brain and are responsible for 20% of all ischemic strokes; 80% of cardioemboli involve the anterior cerebral circulation.

In general, cardioembolic strokes have a worse prognosis and produce larger, more disabling strokes than other ischemic stroke subtypes.

Sources of cardiac emboli (Fig. 5.1) include the following:

1. Atrial fibrillation, which results in thrombus formation in the left atrium

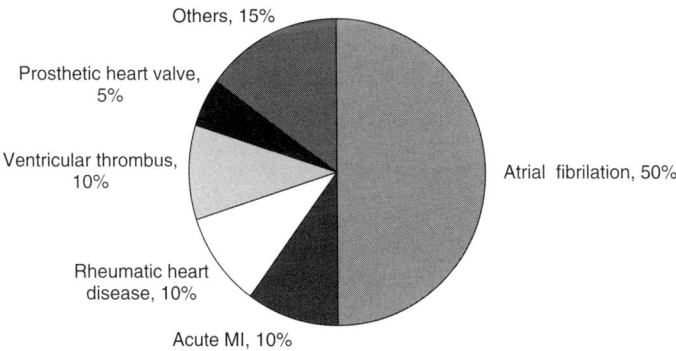

FIGURE 5.1. Sources of cardioembolic stroke.

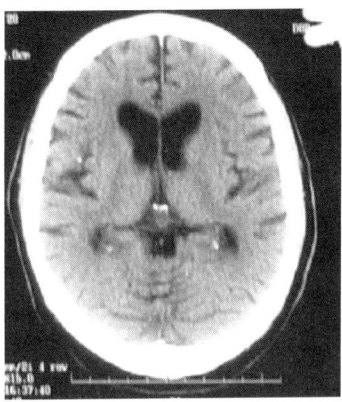

FIGURE 5.2. Calcified embolus in middle cerebral artery territory.

2. Heart valve lesions
3. Acute (<6 weeks) myocardial infarction
4. Mural defects including intracardiac tumors and patent foramen ovale

The composition of cardiac emboli varies, being fibrin in atrial fibrillation, mainly platelets in valve leaflet prolapse and in mitral annulus calcification calcium (Fig. 5.2), and infective vegetations in infective endocarditis.

THE MANAGEMENT OF ATRIAL FIBRILLATION

> **Recommendations**
>
> All patients with atrial fibrillation are at risk of stoke and warfarin anticoagulation should be considered.

Atrial fibrillation (AF) is the commonest arrhythmia. It is classified either as heart valve disease etiology, in particular rheumatic fever, or as nonvalvular disease etiology, which in Western populations is far more common.

In AF the irregularly beating left atrial wall causes blood stasis and thus thrombus formation, which can embolize to the brain. In rheumatic heart disease the atrium is usually enlarged, increasing the risk of blood stasis.

Atrial fibrillation increases with age to 10% in those over 80 years old. The lifetime risk of developing AF after the age of 40 years is 1 in 4. In the United Kingdom that is an incidence of chronic AF in those older than 60 years of 3 per 1000 person years.

Significance

The average absolute risk of stroke in untreated patients with nonvalvular AF is 5% per annum (i.e., a fivefold increase in the risk of stroke compared with those in sinus rhythm) and 12% per annum in patients who have suffered a cerebrovascular event.

A stroke associated with AF carries a higher morbidity and mortality. The risk of stroke in patients with intermittent (paroxysmal) AF is as high as it is for those with established AF. In nonvalvular AF, the risk of stroke is similar in men and women. However, the presence of AF does not always mean it is the cause of a recent cerebrovascular event; other possible causes are present in 20% of fibrillating stroke patients.

MAKING THE DIAGNOSIS OF ATRIAL FIBRILLATION

Clinical Features

Atrial fibrillation is often asymptomatic, especially if it is chronic, but when paroxysmal it is more likely to be associated with the following:

1. Palpitations
2. Chest discomfort

3. Fatigue or light-headedness
4. Fainting
5. Shortness of breath

Investigations

Electrocardiogram (ECG)

Indications. All patients clinically in AF and all patients who have suffered a cerebrovascular event should have an ECG

Findings. In recent-onset AF, the ECG shows rapid irregular f waves at a rate of 350 to 600/minute. Due to the variable conduction through the atrioventricular node, the ventricular electrical response (QRS complex) is irregular. With chronic AF, the f waves are not visible and AF is diagnosed solely by the absence of P waves and the irregular ventricular (QRS complex) response.

Twenty-Four-Hour Electrocardiogram

Indications. The 24-hour ECG is used to catch intermittent runs of AF in patients who give a history suggestive of AF or have suffered a cerebrovascular event.

Findings. Older people have occasional ectopics, and the diagnosis should only be made when sustained runs of AF are recorded.

Echocardiogram

Indications. An echocardiogram should be considered in patients with both of the following:

1. Cardiac abnormalities including AF, heart failure, recent myocardial infarcts, and heart murmurs; and
2. Recent ischemic cerebrovascular events, especially those that appear to be nonlacunar in nature (i.e., arise from a probable extracerebral source).

Actual thrombus is often not detected, but echocardiographic features that suggest the heart as a source of emboli include the following:

1. Left ventricular dysfunction
2. Atrial size over 4.7 cm
3. Atrial or ventricular thrombus
4. Mitral valve disease

If a transesophageal echo is undertaken, added cerebrovascular risk factors include the following:

1. The presence of aortic atheromatous plaque (fourfold)
2. Left atrial appendage thrombus

Treatment

Treatment of Underlying Cause
Before assuming AF is idiopathic, it is important to exclude common causes of AF which include the following:

1. Associated cardiac disease (ischemic heart disease, congestive cardiac failure, mitral valve disease)
2. Thyrotoxicosis
3. Alcohol excess
4. Infections including pneumonia
5. Pulmonary embolus

Treatment to Restore and Maintain Sinus Rhythm
Recent-onset AF reverts spontaneously to sinus rhythm in 50% of patients irrespective of digoxin treatment. If not, the chances of successful cardioversion in recent-onset AF are high if the left atrium is normal. In chronic AF, cardioversion is much less likely to be successful.

Invasive treatments such as ablating the sinoatrial node and then inserting pacing wires do not appear to reduce the risk of thromboembolic events.

It is usually best to just aim to control the heart rate, in hemodynamically stable patients with digoxin in combination with beta-blockers or calcium channel blockers.

The most common drug side effects of digoxin are associated with an overdose and include gastrointestinal disturbances (anorexia, nausea, vomiting, diarrhea, and abdominal cramps), headaches, visual disturbances, fatigue, and confusion.

Treatment to Reduce the Risk of Stroke
The mainstay of treatment of AF to reduce the risk of a cerebrovascular event is warfarin anticoagulation aiming for an international normalized ratio (INR) of 2.0 to 3.0.

Mode of Action. Warfarin acts by inhibiting the carboxylation of several clotting factors in the liver, by inhibiting the vitamin K–dependent carboxylating enzymes.

Treatment Indications

1. Primary prevention (patients with AF but no history of cerebrovascular events): warfarin should be considered for all

patients with atrial fibrillation, but those with no associated risk factors and who are younger than 65 years old can be treated with aspirin alone.

Evidence: Meta-analysis of five large randomized controlled trials has shown a large absolute risk reduction (ARR) in stroke by anticoagulating patients with atrial fibrillation from 4.5% to 1.4% per year with little increase in major bleeds (warfarin 1.2% vs. control 1.0%) including intracranial bleeds (0.3% vs. 0.1%). Meta-analysis of three primary prevention trials have shown that in AF there is an ARR if aspirin is taken of 1.5% (from 5.2% placebo to 3.7% aspirin per year) (Hart et al., 1999, 2003).

2. Secondary prevention (patients with AF and a history of cerebrovascular events): anticoagulation with warfarin aiming for an INR of 2.0 to 3.0.

Evidence: The European Atrial Fibrillation Trial (1993) (EAFT) randomized patients with nonvalvular AF and a recent minor cerebrovascular event to oral anticoagulation or placebo or aspirin. Anticoagulation with warfarin was significantly more effective in reducing the annual incidence of stroke from 12% to 4% per year, even though the incidence of major hemorrhage was higher in this group (2.8% vs. 0.7% in the control group). Aspirin does reduce the risk of stroke in this group but only by an ARR of 2.5% per year (Saxena and Koudstaal, 2004).

Contraindications. Contraindications to warfarin use include severe renal impairment, severe hepatic impairment, severe hypertension, and pregnancy (especially first and third trimesters).

Complications of Warfarin. Maintaining the INR: The dose of warfarin required varies and is difficult to predict. Therefore, the patient needs to be regularly monitored. In the U.K. this is undertaken at large anticoagulation clinics, which interferes with patients' daily activities. Their quality of life is further affected, as fluxes in their intake of alcohol or certain foods such as salads and vegetables can influence the INR reading. If the INR falls below 2.0, the risk of stroke increase. An INR below 1.5 has a 3.5 times greater risk of stroke than one of 2.0, but if it is above 3.0 the risk of bleeding increases.

Bleeding is the most significant complication. This usually occurs into the gastrointestinal tract, brain, or muscle tissues. The risk of bleeding is either drug dependent (dose, type, recently changed dose) or patient dependent (increasing with increasing age, a history of major bleed, and several medical conditions such as hypertension, chronic renal failure, and malignancy).

Other complications of warfarin include dermatitis, alopecia, anorexia, nausea, vomiting, stomach cramps, and very rarely skin necrosis when there is an associated clotting factor deficiency.

Patients need to be treated individually, taking into account their risks of stroke from their AF and associated medical problems, their likelihood of compliance, their stability while walking (more falls, more bleeds), and their wishes.

Open Cardiac Thrombectomy and Valve Replacement

Surgical removal of a large cardiac intramural thrombus is very rarely needed and is almost always associated with another cardiac pathology such as a ventricular aneurysm or valvular lesion.

Bibliography

European Atrial Fibrillation Trial Study Group. Secondary prevention in non-rheumatic atrial fibrillation after transient ischaemic attack or minor stroke. Lancet 1993;342:1255–1262.

Hart RG, Benavente O, McBride R, Pearce LA. Antithrombotic therapy to prevent stroke in patients with atrial fibrillation: a meta-analysis. Ann Intern Med 1999;131:492-501.

Hart R, Halperin JL, Pearce LA, et al. Lessons from the stroke prevention in atrial fibrillation trials. Ann Intern Med 2003;138:831–838.

Saxena R, Koudstaal PJ. Anticoagulants for preventing stroke in patients with non-rheumatic atrial fibrillation and a history of stroke or transient ischaemic attack. Cochrane Database Syst Rev 2004;(1):CD000185.

MANAGING CARDIAC VALVE LESIONS

Several cardiac valve lesions predispose to cardioembolic stroke. The greatest risk comes from the following:

1. Mitral stenosis
2. Mechanical prosthetic heart valves
3. Infective endocarditis

Occasionally a cardioembolic stroke can arise from mitral annular calcification, mitral valve prolapse, and calcified aortic stenosis.

THE MANAGEMENT OF MITRAL VALVE STENOSIS AS A CAUSE OF CARDIOEMBOLIC STROKE

Recommendations

Consider oral anticoagulation for all patients with mitral stenosis, especially those in AF.

Chronic rheumatic heart disease is the commonest cause of mitral stenosis. It is most common in developing countries.

Significance

There is an 18-fold increased incidence of ischemic stroke in patients who have AF and rheumatic valve disease. However, the incidence of rheumatic heart disease in developed countries is rare, and so it has a low attributable risk of stroke. There are no good estimates of absolute stroke rates due to mitral valve stenoses.

Making the Diagnosis of Mitral Stenosis

Clinical Features

Clinical symptoms suggestive of mitral valve stenosis include dyspnea, palpitations, hemoptysis, recurrent bronchitis, and chest pains. Clinical signs suggestive of mitral valve stenosis include atrial fibrillation, a left sternal heave, a diastolic murmur, a loud first heart sound, and an opening snap coming just after the second heart sound.

Investigations

1. Electrocardiogram (ECG) identifies AF and P-mitrale, in which the p wave is notched like the letter M, indicating a large left atrium and right ventricular hypertrophy.
2. Chest x-ray may show a large left atrium, splayed carina, and pulmonary edema.
3. Echocardiography identifies the diastolic pressure drop across the valve as well as estimates the reduced mobility of the anterior cusp. Transesophageal echocardiography identifies left atrial thrombus, the degree of thickening, and calcification of the cusps, and the extent to which the subvalve apparatus is involved.

Treatment

Treatment of Underlying Cause. Penicillin prophylaxis is prescribed against further attacks of acute rheumatic fever, especially when undergoing dental treatment. Fluid retention responds to diuretics. Treat chest infections promptly with appropriate antibiotics. Percutaneous balloon valvuloplasty or open surgical valve replacement treats the underlying condition, but often does not reverse the AF.

Treatment to Reduce the Risk of Stroke. Oral anticoagulation is indicted in the presence of AF, irrespective of the nature or severity of the associated valve disease.

Evidence: Evidence is extrapolated from nonvalvular AF disease, as there are no randomized comparisons of different therapies.

Most anticoagulate patients with mitral stenosis are in sinus rhythm, but especially if a left atrial thrombus is present or there have been previous thromboembolic episodes.

THE MANAGEMENT OF PROSTHETIC HEART VALVES AS A CAUSE OF CARDIOEMBOLIC STROKE

Patients with prosthetic heart valves are at increased risk of arterial thromboembolic events, including stroke.

Significance

The risk of thromboembolic stroke is higher for mechanical than for bioprosthetic (tissue) valves such that mechanical prosthetic valves carry a 3% annual risk of stroke, even in patients receiving anticoagulation, and bioprosthetic valves carry an annual risk rate of <1%.

Stroke risk is higher for prosthetic mitral valves than aortic valves.

Prosthetic heart valves are at risk of infective endocarditis and acting as a source of emboli. They account for one third of all cases of endocarditis, and occur in 3% of patients after valvular heart surgery, with the highest risk in the first 3 months postsurgery. Prosthetic valve endocarditis is five times more common with aortic than with mitral prostheses, and may involve mechanical, xenograft, and homograft valves.

Investigations

Echocardiography is used to record valve function.

Treatment

1. Warfarin anticoagulation reduces the risk of stroke from all mechanical prosthetic heart valve emboli, aiming at an INR of 2.5 to 3.5.
2. Addition of aspirin to warfarin anticoagulation in patients with any type of prosthetic heart valves further reduces the risk of death and systemic thromboembolic events, although there is an increased bleeding tendency.
3. Patients with bioprosthetic valves are anticoagulated for 3 months and then commenced on aspirin.
4. Any patient with AF is considered for oral anticoagulation.

Bibliography

Little SH, Massel DR. Antiplatelet and anticoagulation for patients with prosthetic heart valves. *Cochrane Database Syst Rev* 2003;(4):CD003464.
Lip GYH, Gibbs CR. Anticoagulation for heart failure in sinus rhythm. *Cochrane Database Syst Rev* 2000;(2):CD003336.

THE MANAGEMENT OF INFECTIVE ENDOCARDITIS AS A CAUSE OF CARDIOEMBOLIC STROKE

Infective endocarditis is an infection of the endocardium involving the valves and adjacent structures associated with a 20% mortality. It is rare in the general population, with an incidence of 5 per 100,000 patient years, but has a higher incidence in those with either of the following:

1. Valvular disease, in particular mitral valve prolapse, aortic sclerosis, bicuspid aortic valves, or prosthetic heart valves

2. An increased incidence of bacteremias, as occurs in intra-venous drug abusers, those undergoing cardiac catheteriza-tions, or those with preexisting dental caries.

Bacteremias are also more likely in procedures involving mucosal surfaces such as the upper airways (40%) gastroin-testinal tract (10%), or urology procedures (10%).

Infective endocarditis is associated with streptococci in 60% of cases, a staphylococci in 25% of cases, and a gram-negative bacteria such as salmonella in 10% of cases.

Significance

Emboli fragments from an infected vegetation dislodge in up to 50% of cases. This causes a cardioembolic stroke in 20%.

In 10% of cases, a mycotic aneurysm develops, which leads to a subarachnoid hemorrhage in 5%. Infective endocarditis mortality is higher if there is an associated cardioembolic event (around 60% vs. 20%).

Staphylococcus aureus is the agent producing the highest stroke rate.

Mitral valve endocarditis is the most common source of emboli. Emboli are most likely to occur before starting antimi-crobial therapy, and the risk of emboli decreases with time once appropriate antibiotics have been started. The likelihood of embolization does not differ between mitral valve and aortic valve vegetations (Fig. 5.3), and vegetation size does not predict systemic embolization, although vegetations greater than 1 cm are associated with a poor overall outcome.

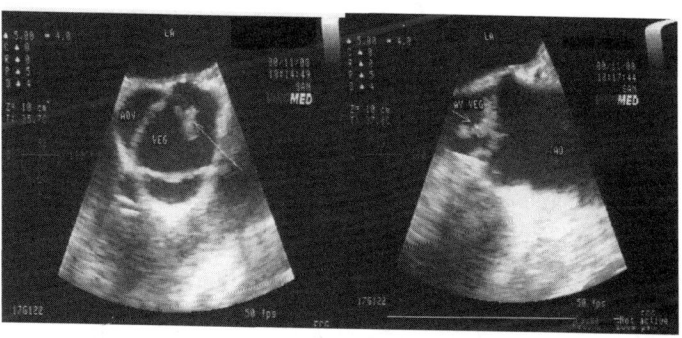

FIGURE 5.3. Aortic valve vegetations.

Making the Diagnosis of Infective Endocarditis

Clinical Features
Infective endocarditis is usually associated with a flu-like illness, with lethargy, fever, and petechial hemorrhages in the subconjunctival, soft palate petechiae, and nail beds (splinter hemorrhages). There can also be painful subcutaneous nodules on the palms or soles (Osler's nodes), and generalized rashes. Patients may also present with painful embolic lesions to the hands or feet, new heart murmurs, and splenomegaly.

Investigations
Blood cultures. If three blood cultures are obtained prior to starting antibiotics, in two thirds of patients they will all be positive.

Echocardiography. Transthoracic echocardiography has a sensitivity of 60% at detecting valvular vegetations, but transesophageal echo has a sensitivity of 90%. Vegetations are missed if they are <2 mm in size.

Magnetic Resonance Imaging. Magnetic resonance imaging (MRI) usually reveals multiple focal areas of ischemia even in the absence of cerebral symptoms.

Treatment

Primary Treatment
Antibiotic prophylaxis to cover is recommended in patients undergoing invasive procedures in which there is an associated risk of a bacteremia and who have known cardiac valve lesions. This usually involves a preprocedural dose of amoxicillin, sometimes with gentamicin.

Evidence: There is little data to confirm its effectiveness or value of antibiotic prophylaxis.

Secondary Treatment
1. Antibiotic therapy reduces the embolic potential when administered in the acute phase. Antibiotics resolve 50% of formed mycotic aneurysms, and decrease, or at least delay, the risk of bleeding from mycotic aneurysms.
   Penicillins, often in combination with gentamicin, are used when the endocarditis is due to susceptible streptococci.
2. Valve surgery is indicated to reduce cardioembolic stroke if a major embolic event has occurred or if the vegetations are >1 cm in diameter. Timing of surgery depends on

whether the stroke results from an embolic infarct or ruptured mycotic aneurysm hemorrhage. In general, if no hemorrhage is detected by computed tomography (CT), surgery is undertaken within 72 hours; if there is a bleed, it is delay for at least 1 week. However, the operative risk is high, and surgery that is performed within a month of the cerebral event carries a mortality of 40%. Other indications for valve surgery include valve failure causing moderate to severe congestive heart failure (New York Heart Association class III or IV), which can occur in the acute phase or several months later, and an endocardial abscess, which can involve the aortic root, valve ring, or ventricular septum.

3. Anticoagulation is contraindicated in patients with native valve endocarditis, because of unacceptable rates of hemorrhagic stroke. In prosthetic valve endocarditis the risk of embolic phenomena is high if the patient is not anticoagulated (50–70% risk).

   Anticoagulation therapy is sometimes continued in patients with prosthetic valves but at a lower INR of 1.5. If neurologic complications are present or if there is brain CT evidence of hemorrhage, anticoagulation therapy is stopped.

Note on Nonbacterial Thrombotic Endocarditis

Nonbacterial thrombotic endocarditis is the formation of a sterile platelet and fibrin thrombi on cardiac wall. It is associated with malignancy especially of the pancreas and lung, and autoimmune diseases such as systemic lupus erythematosus (SLE). It is reported in patients with severe diseases such as septicemia and extensive burns.

Significance

Mitral and aortic valves are affected most commonly, and embolic stroke occurs in more than a third of patients with nonbacterial thrombotic endocarditis

Investigations

Echocardiographic findings include vegetations thickening and regurgitation.

Treatment

Treatment is directed toward control of the underlying disease, and heparin is advocated for stroke prevention. If the patient survives, warfarin is usually then prescribed.

THE MANAGEMENT OF OTHER VALVULAR LESIONS THAT MAY CAUSE CARDIOEMBOLIC STROKE

Native Valve Disease

Indications for Treatment

Oral anticoagulation is indicted in the presence of atrial fibrillation, irrespective of the nature or severity of the associated valve disease. In patients with mitral valve prolapse, anticoagulation to prevent embolization is not required, as the prevalence of mitral valve prolapse is no greater in stroke patients than in the general population, but sometimes aspirin is given.

In patients with mitral regurgitation anticoagulation is indicated in the presence of congestive cardiac failure, marked cardiomegaly with low cardiac output, and an enlarged atrium

In patients with isolated aortic calcified stenosis or bicuspid valves, calcific microemboli can sometimes be detected in the retinal artery, but systemic embolism is uncommon. As the emboli are calcific, anticoagulation is not recommended, and antiplatelet therapy use is empirical.

ACUTE MYOCARDIAL INFARCTION

Recommendations

Assess the risk of cardioembolic stroke following myocardial infarction (MI) in all patients If the risk is high anticoagulation should be considered.

Stroke complicates acute myocardial infarction (MI) in 2% of cases, with most events occurring in the first week post-MI from left ventricular wall mural thromboemboli. An anterior wall MI carries a high risk (5%) of stroke, as 40% of patients with anterior wall MI have left ventricular mural thrombus. This is even higher, (60%), if the MI has resulted in a ventricular aneurysm. Left ventricular thrombi present for more than 3 months will have undergone fibrous organization and are more stable and less likely to embolize.

Atrial fibrillation occurring after an MI is an independent risk factor for stroke. Other causes of stroke following a recent MI include systemic hypotension and iatrogenic causes such as intracerebral hemorrhage secondary to antithrombotic agents, or emboli from catheter thrombus during coronary artery angioplasty or stenting.

Making the Diagnosis

Clinical Features
No individual clinical features predict the likelihood of a mural thrombus formation following MI, but it is more likely in patients with large infarcts, atrial fibrillation, or associated congestive cardiac failure.

Investigations
Echocardiography identifies a left ventricle thrombus. If not found, the presence of a ventricular aneurysm, dilated ventricle, or area of wall motion abnormalities suggests an increased probability of developing thrombus.

Treatment to Reduce Post–Myocardial Infarction Cardioembolic Stroke

Treatment Indications

Formal anticoagulation is not routine following a MI, but is considered in patients at risk of cardioembolism. These include patients who have suffered from the following:

1. Large anterior wall MI
2. MI complicated by severe left ventricular dysfunction
3. Congestive cardiac failure
4. Echocardiographic evidence of mural thrombus or left ventricular aneurysm
5. Previous emboli
6. Atrial fibrillation

Outline of Treatment

Heparin anticoagulation is commenced as soon as possible after the diagnosis of MI has been made. This is followed by oral warfarin anticoagulation for 3 to 6 months, aiming for an INR of 2.5. Antiplatelet treatment is usually continued at the same time. After this period, warfarin is continued in the presence of AF and often in congestive cardiac failure and ventricular aneurysms; in other cases antiplatelet agents alone are used.

Evidence: Low-dose heparin reduces the incidence of mural thrombi in MI patients from 21.9% to 14.2% (p = .03). There is no evidence that thrombolysis alone affects the risk of left ventricular mural thrombosis. Oral anticoagulants in patients who survived MI showed a relative risk reduction (RRR) of stroke of 45% over 3 years, which is significantly greater than the affect of aspirin alone.

Complications and Contraindications of Treatment

The complications and contraindications are the same as for anticoagulation (see above).

Bibliography

Lip GYH, Chin BSP, Prasad N. Antithrombolytic therapy in myocardial infarction and stable angina. In: ABC of Antithrombotic Therapy. London: BMJ Books, 2003:35–37.

MURAL DISEASE

This sectioncovers the following topics:

1. Management of chronic cardiac failure as a cause of cardioembolic stroke
2. Management of the patent foramen ovale (PFO) as a cause of cardioembolic stroke
3. The management of cardiac tumors as a cause of cardioembolic stroke

Management of Chronic Cardiac Failure as a Cause of Cardioembolic Stroke

---

Recommendations

Oral anticoagulation should be considered in chronic cardiac failure when associated with atrial fibrillation (AF), previous thromboembolic events, or fresh unstable left ventricular thrombus.

Chronic cardiac failure is a syndrome usually secondary to ischemic heart disease, hypertension, or idiopathic dilated cardiomyopathy. It is common, with an incidence of 25 per 1000 per year and a prevalence of 1%, which increases with age, reaching 30% in those aged over 80 years. When severe (New York Heart Association [NYHA] class IV), it is associated with a 30% annual mortality rate.

The annual risk of stroke in patients with mild chronic cardiac failure (NYHA class II to III) is 1.5%, and in patents with severe chronic cardiac failure (NYHA class III to IV) it is 4%. In patients with chronic cardiac failure and AF, the risk of stroke is 10% per year, compared with the risk in the general disease-free population of 0.5%.

Making the Diagnosis of Chronic Cardiac Failure

Clinical Features. Common clinical features are fatigue, dyspnea, and ankle edema. Signs of fluid retention such as lung crepitations, raised jugular vein pressure (JVP), and edema may be present, as may signs of impaired perfusion such as cold clammy skin, and signs of ventricular dysfunction such as displaced apex, right ventricular heave, third or fourth heart sound, mitral or tricuspid regurgitation, and tachycardia.

Investigations. The diagnosis of chronic cardiac failure is made on chest radiography, echocardiography, and, in selected cases, cardiac catheterization and radionuclide ventriculography. Echocardiography assesses ventricular dysfunction as left ventricular ejection systolic fraction. This is a strong predictor of the risk of stroke, and those with an ejection fraction less than 28% are at particular risk.

Evidence: For every absolute decrease of 5% in left ventricular ejection fraction (LVEF) the risk of stroke increases 18%.

Echocardiography also identifies left ventricular mural thrombus, and features likely to predispose to thrombus formation, such as ventricular aneurysms, a dilated ventricle, and areas of wall motion dysfunction.

Treatment to Reduce Cardioembolic Stroke

Treatment Indications. Warfarin treatment in chronic cardiac failure is indicated in the presence of AF, previous ischemic strokes, or new or unstable left ventricular mural thrombus. Warfarin treatment should be considered in chronic cardiac failure in the presence of a poor LVEF (<28%), acute left ventricular aneurysms, and idiopathic dilated cardiomyopathies. Warfarin treatment is not indicated in chronic cardiac failure when the patient is in sinus rhythm and has no other risk factors, when there is a chronic left ventricular aneurysm, or when any ventricular mural thrombus is chronic and organized.

Evidence: For warfarin: Evidence reviewed in a Cochrane review, from randomized controlled trials (RCTs), and from observational studies showed a reduction in mortality and cardiovascular events with anticoagulants compared to control. The evidence, however, only supports the use of oral anticoagulation in certain patients with heart failure

For aspirin: Observational trials have shown a beneficial reduction of stroke with aspirin in patients with chronic heart failure, but this is not as great a reduction as warfarin has in preventing strokes in heart failure and may be due to the fact that aspirin has no effect on the risk of systemic embolization in patients with documented left ventricular thrombi.

For doing nothing: Meta-analysis of randomized control trials do not support the routine use of oral anticoagulants in heart failure patients who are in sinus rhythm.

Bibliography

Lip GYH, Chin BSP. Antithrombolytic therapy in chronic heart failure in sinus rhythm. In: ABC of Antithrombotic Therapy. London: BMJ Books, 2003:46–50.

Lip GYH, Gibbs CR. Antiplatelet agents versus control or anticoagulation for heart failure in sinus rhythm. Cochrane Database Syst Rev 2001;(4):CD003333.

Lip GYH, Gibbs CR. Anticoagulation for heart failure in sinus rhythm. Cochrane Database Syst Rev 2001;(4):CD003336.

Management of the Patent Foramen Ovale as a Cause of Cardioembolic Stroke

Recommendations

Consider oral anticoagulation before considering closure techniques.

Cerebrovascular events due to a venous paradoxical embolization through a patent foramen ovale (PFO) are rare. Although it may account for up to 30% of cases when no other cause can be found (cryptogenic stroke), and a PFO is present in 25% of the normal population, in most cases a PFO is a coincidental finding.

Paradoxical embolism from the venous side causing stroke via other routes such as ventricular septal defects and pulmonary arteriovenous fistulae are even rarer.

Clinical Features

There are no reliable diagnostic criteria to confirm a cerebrovascular event is due to paradoxical emboli. However, it is more likely in the following situations:

1. In young patients
2. When associated with recent acute migraine
3. When there is evidence of a venous embolic source
4. When there are associated factors that may increase the right heart pressure
   a. When Valsalva manoeuvre or cough occurred just prior to the stroke
   b. In regular divers
   c. Occurring during air travel
5. Posterior cerebral artery infarcts are more common than anterior ones.

Investigations
Contrast transesophageal echocardiography is the best investigation to assess the presence and severity of a PFO.

PFO factors associated with a higher cerebrovascular recurrence rate are as follows:

1. Large sized PFO (>5 mm)
2. Severe right to left shunting (>50% left atrium filling)
3. An associated interseptal aneurysm

Management
Treatment options include the following:

1. Open surgical closure repair
2. Percutaneous transcatheter closure
3. Medical treatment (either antiplatelet or anticoagulant therapy)
4. No treatment

There are no good prospective trials to suggest the most appropriate means of managing patients who have suffered a cerebrovascular event believed to be due to a paradoxical embolization through a PFO. Currently, antithrombotic treatment is considered first line, and closure techniques are considered in patients with recurrent cerebrovascular events despite medical management, or when there is definite evidence of paradoxical embolization.

Bibliography
Khiani R, Sastry S, Heagerty AM, Gamble E, McCollum CN. Antithrombotic treatment for preventing recurrent stroke due to paradoxical embolism. Cochrane Database Syst Rev 2002;(3):CD004432.

The Management of Cardiac Tumors as a Cause of Cardioembolic Stroke
Cardiac myxomas are benign, 3- to 10-cm polypoidal tumors arising from a stalk usually of the left atrium that do not locally invade and rarely metastase. They occur in 2 per 100,000 in the general population, more often in women (2:1), and usually between 30 and 60 years of age.

Significance
Systemic emboli occur in 40% and are frequently the first manifestation of disease. Of these 80% are cerebrovascular emboli.

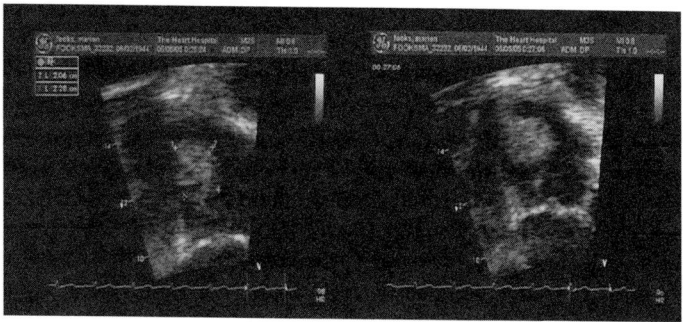

FIGURE 5.4. Atrial myxoma. A rare cause of cerebral emboli. The diagnosis is made on echocardiography, identifying an echo dense mobile mass within the atrium.

Making the Diagnosis

Clinical Features. Myxomas are usually asymptomatic until they embolize or get very large and present with symptoms of left atrial obstruction, for example, progressive breathlessness, orthopnea, paroxysmal nocturnal dyspnea, fluid retention, and atrial arrhythmias.

Investigations. Echocardiography makes the diagnosis by identifying an echo dense mobile mass within the atrium restrained only by a peduncle (Fig. 5.4). An ECG and chest x-ray are of no help, and angiography is not necessary as it adds no further information.

Treatment

The tumor is surgically removed, with a full-thickness button of normal atrial septal tissue around the tumor base. The resulting defect is usually repaired with a small patch. The surgical risk is low, functional results are good, and recurrence is rare.

Chapter 6

Reducing Cervical Vessel Embolic Events

THE MANAGEMENT OF CAROTID ARTERY ATHEROSCLEROTIC STENOSIS

Recommendations

1. Patients with carotid artery bifurcation stenosis of >70% who have suffered an appropriate nondisabling cerebrovascular event and are likely to live for more than 6 months should be considered for a carotid endarterectomy as soon as possible.
2. Carotid stenting should only be considered within the confines of a trial.
3. Carotid surgery for a >70% asymptomatic stenosis should be considered, but with appropriate assessment of the risks and benefits.

Atherosclerotic stenoses tend to develop at the common carotid artery bifurcation into the internal and external carotid arteries. This may be due to a flow disturbance. Rupture of this plaque showers emboli into the cerebral circulation.

Significance

In patients who have had a cerebrovascular event, carotid artery stenosis is a strong predictor of subsequent stroke. The tighter the stenosis, the greater the risk of subsequent stroke. With extreme stenosis (>90%) the annual risk of ipsilateral ischemic stroke is about 20%; and with stenosis of 80% to 89% it is 15%; and with stenosis of 70% to 79%, is it 6% to 10%.

If the patient remains asymptomatic without intervention following an initial cerebrovascular event, the risk of stroke falls off exponentially over 2 to 3 years.
Although it has been claimed that up to one third of these strokes are due to intracranial small-vessel disease (lacunar) or embolism from the heart, and thus not to be prevented by carotid endarterectomy, following surgery the annual risk of stroke falls to 1% per year. In asymptomatic patients with carotid stenoses >70%, the risk of any stroke is 3% per year, and the risk of an ipsilateral ischemic stroke is 2%. This may be higher in tight stenoses >90%.

MAKING THE DIAGNOSIS OF A CAROTID ARTERY STENOSIS

Clinical Features
The clinical features of a carotid territory cerebrovascular event (Fig. 2.2) are not always easy to elucidate, as there is considerable intraclinician variation, and the features are not always associated with a carotid stenosis.

Neck Bruit
There is a correlation between neck bruits and the severity of the carotid stenosis; however, a bruit is not sufficiently sensitive or specific enough to actually make the diagnosis, because a bruit is often absent at the extremes of stenosis and if present may be a consequence of other flow disturbances such as an external carotid artery stenosis, or a hyperdynamic circulation as occurs in thyrotoxicosis, pregnancy, and anemia. The bruit may be transmitted from the heart and great vessels

Carotid Artery Atherosclerosis
Carotid artery atherosclerosis is more likely if other vascular beds are also affected as in those with ischemic heart disease or peripheral arterial disease or when the patient has several cerebrovascular risk factors.

Investigations

Carotid Artery Duplex Scanning
Indications All patients with transient ischemic attack (TIA) or stroke should be evaluated for a carotid artery stenosis. Those with nondisabling carotid ischemic cerebrovascular events should be given priority, and urgent carotid surgical intervention could

be considered if there is an appropriate stenosis. In patients with noncarotid or disabling carotid cerebrovascular events, a scan is indicated to help determine the cause of stroke and plan appropriate prevention.

Advantages The procedure is accurate, quick, inexpensive, and noninvasive. The accuracy of defining internal carotid artery origin stenosis and plaque characteristics is such that most surgeons are usually prepared to undertake surgery without further carotid artery imaging.

Disadvantages The scanning is operator dependent and therefore often not reproducible.

Angiography

Indications The indications are decreasing, as angiography is being replaced by duplex ultrasound alone. Angiography is used when heavy calcification obscures the duplex ultrasound assessment of the degree of stenosis at the carotid bifurcation, or when an intracerebral lesion is suspected, such as cerebral aneurysms, arteriovenous malformations, and arteritis.

Advantages Angiography offers images of very good quality. The symptomatic carotid surgery trials are based on angiography.

Disadvantages

1. Angiography only images the lumen of the vessel and not the wall.
2. It does not give plaque morphology information.
3. Risks of the procedure relate to the following:
   a. The contrast medium (such as allergic reaction, and worsening of renal failure especially in diabetics)
   b. Catheter disrupting atheroma plaque, resulting in either distal embolization and precipitating a stroke (0.5–4%) or vessel wall dissection
   c. Catheter puncture site hematoma

Computed Tomographic Angiography

Indications As computerized software images improve, this method of investigation is likely to become more common. It has replaced angiography.

Advantages Computed tomographic angiography (CTA) is much less invasive and quicker than angiography. It uses less contrast material and is therefore considered safer.
It is more accurate than magnetic resonance angiography (MRA) at determining the degree of vessel stenosis.

Disadvantages

1. No information on plaque morphology
2. Risks are associated with the side effects of contrast material

Magnetic Resonance Angiography

Indications Magnetic resonance angiography (MRA) is undertaken to view extra- and intracerebral vessels when reliable duplex ultrasound is not available or a preoperative confirmation of vessel stenosis is required. A vessel dissection is indicated from the duplex ultrasound.

Disadvantages

1. MRA images are not as clear as angiographic images and therefore not as accurate at determining degrees of stenosis.
2. Claustrophobia
3. A metal implant may be affected by the strong magnetic field.
4. If the implant is close to the examination site. it is difficult to get high-quality images.

Treatment

Carotid Endarterectomy

Outline of Procedure Under local or general anesthesia, the carotid vessels are exposed and clamped on either side of the bifurcation and stenosis. A plastic tube or shunt is used to provide blood to the brain if indicated by either an alteration in neurology on cross-clamping or alteration in a secondary marker such as carotid artery stump pressure or electromyography (EMG) recordings. The atherosclerotic plaque is then removed and the vessel closed using a synthetic or vein patch. The patient is discharged within 48 hours.

Treatment Indications

Asymptomatic Carotid Stenosis Carotid endarterectomy significantly reduces the risk of stroke in neurologically asymptomatic patients, but the net benefit is low and should only be considered in carefully selected patients.
Evidence: A reduction in the risk of stroke from 3.1% per year to 2.5% per year.

Symptomatic Carotid Stenosis Surgery is indicated in the following patients:

1. Those who have recently experienced a nondisabling cerebrovascular event (the sooner, the better, and if possible within 2 weeks for transient ischemic attacks [TIAs])

2. Those who have an internal carotid artery origin, or common carotid artery stenosis of between 70% and 99%.
3. Those who have a general prognosis of living a year.

Evidence: Carotid endarterectomy reduces the risk of stroke from 8.8% per year to 4.6% per year, an absolute risk reduction (ARR) of 4.2%, with a number to treat of 24 to prevent one stroke per year.

Complications of Treatment
Perioperative Stroke Carotid endarterectomy is associated with an increased relative risk of disabling stroke or death of 2.5. The risk of stroke is not related to the degree of stenosis, but to the surgeon and the patient. Such factors include female gender, hypertension, peripheral arterial disease, and an occluded contralateral internal carotid artery.

Other Perioperative Complications

1. Wound infection (1%)
2. Major neck hematoma (5%)
3. Cranial and peripheral nerve palsies (7%)

CAROTID ARTERY STENTING

Outline of Procedure
An angioplasty balloon dilates the carotid artery stenosis, and then a stent is inserted through the lesion. Atheromatous plaque that is dislodged during the procedure is captured by a distal cerebral protection device, such as a balloon or retractable filter basket placed in the distal internal carotid artery.

Indications for Treatment

Symptomatic Patients
Carotid stenting should be considered within the confines of randomized control trials or in patients not suitable for carotid endarterectomy, such as postradiotherapy carotid stenosis or high-placed stenoses not accessible to open surgery.

Evidence: Cochrane Database meta-analysis of the few randomized control trials suggests no significant difference between the odds of death or any stroke at 30 days post–carotid endarterectomy or stenting. There is, however, not sufficient data to provide accurate estimates of the risk and effectiveness of the procedure. Two more recent randomized studies (Stent Protection Angioplasty versus Carotid Endarterectomy [SPACE] and Endarterectomy versus stenting in patients with severe symptomatic stenosis trial [EVA]-35) found carotid endarterectomy to be superior to stenting.

Asymptomatic Patients
Carotid stenting should be considered within the confines of a trial.

Evidence: Evidence is sparse and extrapolated from asymptomatic carotid surgery trials.

Complications of Treatment

Periprocedure Stroke
The risk of periprocedure disabling stroke and death within 30 days is 6% in randomized trials, which is the same as for carotid endarterectomy.

Other Perioperative Complications
There are significantly few cranial nerve palsies compared with carotid endarterectomy. The hematoma rate at the groin requiring open surgery or prolonging the hospital stay is not significantly different from that occurring surgically in the neck.

How Well Is Carotid Artery Stenosis Managed at Present?
Despite carotid endarterectomy being subjected to more randomized control trials than any other surgical technique and having been shown to be an effective form of treatment in selected patients, the aim to improve outcomes and reduce the perceived associated morbidity of surgery has resulted in many centers outside the U.K. undertaking carotid artery stenting despite the "current evidence not supporting a widespread change in clinical practice away from recommending carotid endarterectomy as the treatment of choice for suitable carotid artery stenosis".

Bibliography
CAVATAS investigators. Endovascular versus surgical treatment in patients with carotid stenosis in the Carotid and Vertebral Artery Transluminal Angioplasty Study (CAVTAS): randomized trial. Lancet 2001;357:1729–1737.

Chambers BR, You RX, Donnan GA. Carotid endarterectomy for asymptomatic carotid stenosis. Cochrane Database Syst Rev 2005;(2):CD001923.

Cina CS, Clase CM, Haynes RB. Carotid endarterectomy for symptomatic carotid stenosis. Cochrane Database Syst Rev 1999;(3):CD001081.

Coward LJ, Featherstone RL, Brown MM. Percutaneous transluminal angioplasty and stenting for carotid artery stenosis. Cochrane Database Syst Rev 2004;(1):CD000515.

Mas J-L, Chatellier G, et al. Endarterectomy versus stenting in patients with severe symptomatic stenosis. N Engl J Med 2006;355:1660–1667.

SPACE Collaborators. Stent Protection Angioplasty versus Carotid Endarterectomy in symptomatic patients: 30 days results from the SPACE Trial. Lancet 2006;368:1239–1247.

THE MANAGEMENT OF CAROTID ARTERY DISSECTION

Recommendations

Consider anticoagulation as part of secondary prevention.

Dissection of the carotid artery occurs between the media and adventitia, creating a false lumen leading to stenosis, occlusion, or a pseudoaneurysm, and any resulting thrombus can embolize. Associated cerebrovascular events may thus have a hemodynamic or embolic origin. Intracranial dissections can lead to a subarachnoid hemorrhage.

Incidence
The incidence is 2 to 3/100,000 per year.

Significance
Extracranial internal carotid artery dissection is responsible for 2.5% of all strokes, being the second leading cause of stroke in patients under 45 years of age. A cerebrovascular event occurs in 65% of carotid dissections. The 10-year dissection recurrence rate is 11%, with the greatest risk during the first month and then about 1% risk per year. The stroke recurrence rate is 3%.

Making the Diagnosis

Clinical Features
Clinical presentation is varied, requiring a high index of suspicion, but more common presentations are as follows:

1. Headache: constant, stabbing, piercing, or throbbing, including facial and neck pain on the same side as the dissection, usually preceding a cerebrovascular event, (unlike a headache associated with stroke, which usually follows the cerebrovascular event).
2. Oculosympathetic paresis: Horner syndrome (50%) is probably due to the sudden enlargement of the internal carotid artery affecting the overlying sympathetic fibers.
3. Cranial nerve palsies (10%)
4. Predisposing carotid artery trauma: for example, blunt trauma, as occurs with neck manipulations by chiropractors, and intraoral trauma by foreign bodies such, as falling on one's face while a pencil is in one's mouth.

5. Occasionally there is an underlying predisposing connective tissue disorder such as Marfan syndrome or Ehlers-Danlos syndrome type IV.

Investigations

Duplex scanning Duplex scanning is used early to make the diagnosis. Findings include a high-resistance waveform, a double lumen, an intimal flap, vessel occlusion, or a long tapered stenosis narrowing with intima overlying intramural thrombus.

Magnetic Resonance Imaging and Angiography Magnetic resonance imaging (MRI) identifies the dissection as a vessel mural hematoma. Magnetic resonance angiography (MRA) shows irregularities, narrowings, and aneurysmal dilations of the dissected vessels.

Angiography Findings include a double lumen and intimal flap, a string sign with long tapered narrowing, segmental stenosis or occlusion, membrane or flap, and multiple scalloped narrowing

Transcranial Doppler Ultrasonography Transcranial Doppler (TCD) ultrasonography can detect intracranial arterial abnormalities, provide information on collateral flow, and follow microemboli in the middle cerebral artery distal to a carotid dissection. The presence of emboli on TCD scans correlates with stroke risk.

Treatment

Primary Prevention This disorder is rare, and even in high-risk groups primary prevention is not indicated.

Secondary Prevention Either warfarin anticoagulation or anti-platelet drugs are prescribed.

Evidence: There are no RCTs to determine the best form of therapy. Ligation of the carotid artery with or without extracranial-intracranial bypass and arterial reconstruction is reserved for progressive cases where a worsening stroke has been proven on transcranial Doppler to be due to carotid emboli. It is very rarely undertaken.

Evidence: There are no RCTs.

Bibliography

Lyrer P, Engelter S. Antithrombotic drugs for carotid artery dissection. Cochrane Database Syst Rev 2003;(1):CD000255.

THE MANAGEMENT OF VERTEBROBASILAR ARTERY AND INTRACRANIAL ARTERY ATHEROSCLEROTIC STENOSES

Recommendations

1. Treat patients with suspected intracranial artery stenoses with antiplatelet therapy.
2. Apply general cardiovascular risk factor management.

Twenty-five percent of ischemic strokes occur in the vertebrobasilar arterial area. Vertebral artery stenosis affects both the extra- and intracranial vessels.

Significance

Intracranial artery stenoses secondary to atherosclerosis are responsible for 5% to 10% of all ischemic strokes. The annual risk of stroke in patients with intracranial artery stenosis is 3% to 15%. Those at highest risk are patients with severe vertebrobasilar artery stenoses and recurrent cerebrovascular events on antithrombotic therapy. Patients with symptomatic intracranial vertebrobasilar artery stenosis are also at risk of other cardiovascular events

Making the Diagnosis of Vertebrobasilar Stenosis

Clinical Features

The clinical features of a vertebrobasilar territory cerebrovascular event (Fig. 2.2) are not always easy to elucidate, as there is considerable variation.

Investigations

1. Transcranial Doppler ultrasound (TCD) suggests the presence of stenoses by variations in peak systolic velocity reading.
2. Magnetic resonance angiography (MRA) suggests the presence of intracranial stenoses.
3. Catheter angiography is diagnostic, but should be reserved for those in whom intracranial stenoses are likely, and invasive intervention is a consideration.

Treatment

Primary Prevention There is no evidence that treating asymptomatic vertebrobasilar artery stenoses, be they extra- or intracranial, prophylactically protect against stroke.

Secondary Prevention

1. Antithrombotic therapy is the mainstay of treatment for intracranial stenoses. Most patients are treated with antiplatetlets, as warfarin adds no benefit and has greater side effects.
2. Surgery is restricted to stenosis localized to the origin of the vertebral artery at the subclavian artery, and involves either vertebral endarterectomy or transposition to the common carotid artery. It is rarely undertaken in the U.K. despite retrospective studies suggesting good technical results (procedural stroke or death rate 3% with a 90% 10-year patency).

Vertebral Basilar Intracranial Stenosis Angioplasty and Stenting
This form of intervention is gaining momentum in Europe, despite the fact that the evidence for this treatment is based only on small retrospective open-labeled case series with very short follow-up periods and a 3% to 40% rate of stroke or death during or after angioplasty.

How Well Are Intracranial Artery Stenosis Managed?
Most centers do not investigate for intracranial artery stenoses. Most patients are treated with antiplatelet therapy anyway, and while evidence for the benefits of stent angioplasty is lacking, it is only considered in very few units. This is likely to change with new trials underway.

Bibliography

Chimowitz MI, Lynn MJ, Howlett-Smith H, et al., for the Warfarin–Aspirin Symptomatic Intracranial Disease Trial Investigators. Comparison of warfarin and aspirin for symptomatic intracranial arterial stenosis. N Engl J Med 2005;352:1305–1316.

Coward LJ, Featherstone RL, Brown MM. Percutaneous transluminal angioplasty and stenting for vertebral artery stenosis. Cochrane Database Syst Rev 2005;(2):CD000516.

Cruz-Flores S, Leacock RO, Diamond AL. Angioplasty for intracranial artery stenosis. Cochrane Database Syst Rev 2002;(4):CD004133.

THE MANAGEMENT OF AORTIC ARCH ATHEROSCLEROTIC EMBOLI

> **Recommendations**
>
> Do not forget the arch as a source of emboli and consider anticoagulation as part of secondary prevention.

Significance

There is a statistical link between the presence of atherosclerotic disease in the aortic arch and ischemic stroke. The highest risk of ischemic stroke is associated with plaques >4 mm in the proximal arch, which is an independent risk factor even with the presence of carotid stenosis and atrial fibrillation. The annual risk of recurrent ischemic stroke is 12% per year in patients with aortic arch plaques >4 mm. The risk of stroke, myocardial infarction (MI), peripheral embolism, and vascular events is 26% per year. The presence of aortic arch atheroma is a significant intraoperative risk for stroke while undergoing cardiac surgery.

Investigations

Transesophageal echocardiography detects plaques in the aortic arch. It is accurate, safe, and well tolerated.

Treatment

Oral anticoagulants, antiplatelet agents, and surgery to remove the plaque have all been suggested, but there are no studies that clearly identify the superiority treatment.

The Aortic Arch Cerebral Hazards (ARCH) trial is underway comparing different treatments.

Part III

Reducing the Risk of Stroke
by Modifying Atherosclerotic
Risk Factors

Chapter 7
Managing Hypertension

Recommendations

Control blood pressure to ensure it is less than 130/80 mm Hg.

The American heart association defines hypertension as follows:

1. A systolic blood pressure >140 mm Hg or a diastolic blood pressure >90 mm Hg.
2. The taking of antihypertensive medicines.
3. A patient being told by a health professional on two occasions that the patient has high blood pressure.

A higher percentage of men than women have hypertension up to the age of 55; thereafter the prevalence is equal. It is higher in women taking the oral contraceptive pill and higher in blacks than in whites.

SIGNIFICANCE
Hypertension is a major treatable independent risk factor for stroke. There is a graded relationship between diastolic pressure and stroke, with the risk of stroke rising steadily as diastolic pressure level rises even in the normal range; that is, the incidence of stroke increases by 46% for every 7.5 mm Hg increase in diastolic pressure such that when the blood pressure is above 160/90 the risk is four times greater than for those with normal blood pressure.

All measures of raised blood pressure (systolic, diastolic, and pulse pressure) are associated with an increased incidence of stroke. There is no threshold blood pressure level below which the risk becomes stable. Hypertension is a similar risk factor for stroke due to large-vessel disease, cardioembolic stroke, and lacunae strokes.

Importantly, randomised trials have shown that reducing elevated blood pressure reduces the risk of stroke.

MAKING THE DIAGNOSIS OF HYPERTENSION

Clinical Features
Hypertension is clinically silent, and features of end-organ damage including stroke are long-term manifestations.

Investigations

Measuring Blood Pressure
Conventional manometers with appropriate bladder cuff sizes should be used. The cuff is deflated slowly. Systolic blood pressure is assessed by palpation before auscultation. The diastolic pressure is noted when the sounds (phase V) disappear. The systolic and diastolic pressures should be recorded to the nearest 2 mm Hg. During each visit at least two blood pressure recordings should be made. If they are both high, the blood pressure should be taken on at least four separate visits. If there is any question about an elevated blood pressure, a 24-hour recording can be made.

Hypertensive end-organ damage should be assessed with funduscopy, an electrocardiogram (ECG), and an echocardiogram.

TREATMENT

Who Should Be Treated?

Primary Prevention
All patients found to be hypertensive should be considered for treatment.

Evidence: An overview of 14 treatment trials in 37,000 hypertensive patients concluded that an average blood pressure reduction of 5.8 mm Hg resulted in a 42% reduction in stroke incidence.

Secondary Prevention
Treating hypertension reduces the risk of further cerebrovascular events. All patients who have suffered a cerebrovascular event should be considered for antihypertensive treatment even if their blood pressure is within considered normal values.

Evidence: Even small reductions in blood pressure can have a large reduction in stroke risk. A 5 mm Hg reduction in diastolic blood pressure and 10 mm Hg reduction of systolic blood pressure for 2 years results in a relative risk reduction (RRR) of stroke of 30%.

In the preventing strokes by lowering blood pressure (PROGRESS) trial, which randomized patients who had suffered cerebrovascular events to perindopril and indapamide or controls, a benefit was obtained by patients in the treatment group across the whole spectrum of entry blood pressure, including those with normal blood pressures.

How Should Blood Pressure Be Controlled?
Hypertension should be treated by a combination of lifestyle alterations and medications.

Lifestyle Changes
Dietary advice to reduce salt intake, lose weight, and possibly increase fish oil intake will reduce blood pressure a few mm Hg, but these changes are often difficult to undertake even in motivated patients. There is no good evidence to support the idea that reducing alcohol intake affects the blood pressure. However, exercise can lead to a reduction in blood pressure.

Medications
There are a large number of medications that successfully lower blood pressure and have been shown to reduce cerebrovascular events. These include diuretics, beta-blockers, calcium channel antagonists, angiotensin-converting enzyme (ACE) inhibitors, and angiotension II antagonists. The greater the blood pressure reduction, the greater the stroke risk reduction. There are no class differences on the effect lowered blood pressure has on reducing cardiovascular, including cerebrovascular events.

Evidence: In a meta-analysis considering seven sets of prospectively designed overviews with data from 29 randomized trials (n = 162,341), no significant differences in total major cardiovascular events between regimens based on ACE inhibitors, calcium antagonists, or diuretics or beta-blockers was found.

Complications of Treatment

General Side Effects
Antihypertensive drugs are associated with postural hypotension especially in the aged, which results in falls with associated leg and arm bone fractures, loss of confidence, and ultimately loss of independence.

Specific Side Effects

Thiazide diuretics can induce hypokalemia, and have adverse effect on serum lipid levels, blood glucose, and uric acid levels. Beta-blockers can adversely affect glucose intolerance and lipid metabolism. The ACE inhibitors produce a cough, and a worsening of renal failure in the presence of renal artery stenosis. Calcium channel antagonists can induce ankle swelling and flushing.

How Well Is Hypertension Controlled?

Hypertension is generally not well controlled. Of people who have hypertension, 30% do not know they have it, 34% are on medication and are well controlled, 25% are on medication but not well controlled, 11% are not on medication. Two thirds of first-time stroke patients have a blood pressure above 160/90.

Bibliography

Blood Pressure Lowering Treatment Trialists' Collaboration. Effects of different blood-pressure-lowering regimens on major cardiovascular events: results of prospectively-designed overviews of randomised trials. Lancet 2003;362(9395):1527.

Collins R, Peto R, MacMahon S, et al. Blood pressure, stroke, and coronary heart disease. Part 2, short-term reductions in blood pressure: overview of randomised drug trials in their epidemiological context. Lancet 1990;335:82738.

Staessen J, et al. Cardiovascular protection and blood pressure control a meta-analysis. Lancet 2001;358:1305.

Chapter 8
Managing Diabetes

Recommendations

1. Treat all diabetics to obtain a normal fasting plasma glucose (blood sugar) and hemogobin (HbA$_{1c}$) of less than 7%.
2. Use an angiotensin-converting enzyme inhibitor antihypertensive medication.
3. Aggressively control other cerebrovascular risk factors.

The incidence of diabetes continues to increase, with a prevalence of 7% for age-adjusted adults. Diabetes is more common in the Indian subcontinent and Afro-Caribbean communities. Ninety percent of diabetic patients have type 2 diabetes and 40% of people over the age of 40 have "prediabetes," a condition that raises the risk of developing type 2 diabetes, stroke, and ischemic heart disease.

SIGNIFICANCE

Diabetes is an independent risk factor for stroke as well as other atherosclerotic vascular diseases. It is associated with a threefold increased risk of stroke. This is independent of other cerebrovascular risks often associated with diabetes, such as hypertension, obesity, and hyperlipidemia.

Stroke in diabetic patients is more likely in women than in men and is more likely to be fatal. The risk of a recurrent stroke is five fold greater in diabetics than in nondiabetics.

Diabetes is associated with more ischemic small-vessel strokes (36%) than large-vessel strokes (29%) or cardioembolic strokes (28%).

MAKING THE DIAGNOSIS OF DIABETES

Clinical Features

There is no clear correlation between the duration of diabetes and the likelihood and severity of stroke. However, certain complications of diabetes such as diabetic retinopathy and microalbinuria are associated with an increased incidence of stroke. The more severe these complications, the higher the incidence of stroke. Diabetic autonomic neuropathy is another marker of a raised risk of stroke such that an orthostatic blood pressure drop of 10 mm Hg doubles the risk of stroke associated with a sympathetic diabetic neuropathy.

Treatment

The aim of managing diabetes to prevent stroke is twofold: first, to control the blood glucose; and second, to control cerebrovascular risk factors (73% of adults with diabetes have a blood pressure greater than 130/80).

Control Blood Glucose

The treatment aim is to achieve near-normal fasting plasma glucose or as indicated by near-normal hemoglobin Hb1Ac.

Initially this is treated with diet and exercise, and the second-line therapy is usually with oral hypoglycemic drugs such as sulfonylureas and/or metformin, with ancillary acarbose and thiazolidinediones.

Third-line therapy involves insulin.

Evidence: Tight control of blood glucose probably reduces the risk of stroke. If the type 2 diabetes is controlled with hypoglycemic drugs, metformin is recommended.
Evidence: In the UKPDS33 trial, type 2 diabetics with tightly controlled blood glucose levels with sulfonylureas or insulin had fewer microvascular complication (but not macrovascular ones) The UKPDS34 study showed that in obese type 2 diabetics, intensive blood glucose control with metformin had a 5% to 10% reduced combined stroke, myocardial infarction, and death rate when compared with tight control using other hypoglycemic drugs. However, in neither of these studies was stroke an independent consideration.

Aggressive Management of Other Cerebrovascular Risk Factors

Hyperlipidemia An aggressive approach to lower blood cholesterol levels is recommended, as diabetic patients have higher baseline risk levels than nondiabetics matched for age and cardiovascular disease rather than the management having a specific benefit for diabetics over non diabetics.

Evidence: In the Heart Protection Study, diabetic subanalysis showed that simvastatin taken by diabetic patients produced an absolute risk reduction (ARR) of 1.5% in stroke, but that this was no different from nondiabetics (ARR 1.4%). There was similary no difference between diabetic and nondiabetic patients in the number of overall vascular events prevented by reducing cholesterol levels by taking statins (ARR 4.9% vs. 5.6% in diabetic vs. non diabetic subgroups).

Blood Pressure Control and Angiotensin-Converting Enzyme Inhibitor Use It is recommended that all diabetics be on an angiotensin-converting enzyme inhibitor (ACE-I) such as ramipril.

Evidence: ACE-I antihypertensives appear, in diabetics in particular, to have a cardioprotective role even in normotensive patients. This includes a reduction in the number of subsequent strokes.

The diabetic arm of the Heart Outcomes Prevention Evaluation Study (HOPE) showed that the addition of an ACE-I to the current medical regimen in patients with vascular disease and diabetes significantly lowered the risk, over 5 years, of myocardial infarction, stroke, or cardiovascular death. For stroke this was an ARR of 1.9% (4.2% vs. 6.1%) and for transient ischemic attacks (TIAs) 1.5% (4.4% vs. 5.9% for treatment vs. placebo). Although the blood pressure was statistically lowered by treatment, it was usually by less than 2 mm Hg.

Bibliography

Mankovsy B, Ziegler D. Stroke in patients with diabetes mellitus. Diabetes Metab Res Rev 2004;20:268–287.

Stettler C, Allemann S, Jüni P, et al. Glycemic control and macrovascular disease in types 1 and 2 diabetes mellitus: Meta-analysis of randomized trials. Am Heart J 2006;152(1):27–38.

Chapter 9
Managing Hyperlipidemia

Recommendations

Raised serum cholesterol levels >3.5 mmol/l should be treated with a statin in patients with

1. Prior cerebrovascular events
2. Other risks of cardiovascular and cerebrovascular death:
   a. Coronary heart disease
   b. Occlusive disease of noncoronary arteries
   c. Diabetes mellitus
   d. Hypertension

SIGNIFICANCE

There is a clear relationship between serum lipid levels and atherosclerosis, with disease progression being directly related to cholesterol and low-density lipoprotein (LDL) levels and inversely related to high-density lipoprotein (HDL) serum levels. The average total cholesterol level is a mean of 5.53 mmol/L (standard deviation [SD] 1.16), but for men and women over 45 years of age, the average is 6.2 mmol/L, which makes the United Kingdom population one of the highest average cholesterol levels in the world. Cerebrovascular and other vascular events are reduced by treating patients at risk even if the total cholesterol is within normal values (>3.5 mmol/L).

MAKING THE DIAGNOSIS OF HYPERLIPIDEMIA

Clinical Features

Clinical features are usually confined to recognized hyperlipidemic syndromes (Fredrickson syndromes I to V) and include eruptive xanthoma (yellow papules on the extensor surfaces of back, arms, buttocks, and legs), hepatosplenomegaly, lipemia retinalis (retinal arteries and veins appearing white on funduscopy), xanthelasma, and corneal arcus, although their significance is not clear.

Other causes of hyperlipidemia that need to be identified include the following:

1. Metabolic causes: diabetes mellitus/metabolic syndrome X, hypothyroidism, obesity
2. Renal diseases
3. Drugs including alcohol excess, thiazide diuretics, and corticosteroids.

Investigations

Although there are several components to the lipid profile that can be measured it is common to consider the following:

1. Total serum cholesterol levels using nonfasting samples. This is a simple and reliable test, but can be misleading if there is a raised LDL and reduced HDL cholesterol levels.
2. The LDL serum cholesterol levels are the main laboratory test on which most clinical decisions are made. A fasting sample is required for an accurate result.
3. The HDL cholesterol levels are inversely related to the risk of adverse cardiovascular events. The total serum cholesterol/HDL cholesterol ratio is used in the vascular risk prediction charts.
4. Plasma triglycerides probably have a significant effect on cardiovascular disease, but are only assessed after cholesterol levels are considered from a fasting sample.

TREATMENT

Statin Therapy

Treatment Indications

Raised serum cholesterol levels >3.5 mmol/L should be treated with a statin in patients with either prior cerebrovascular events or other risks of cardiovascular and cerebrovascular death, including coronary heart disease, peripheral vascular disease, diabetes mellitus, or hypertension.

A low dose is initially used. Serum cholesterol levels are checked at 3 weeks, usually with serum liver functions enzyme levels and creatinine kinase levels. Assuming no side effects, the dose is then increased if indicated.

The patient will need to remain on treatment lifelong.

The period between checking cholesterol levels increases as a stable low level is achieved.

Mode of Action

Statins act by inhibiting 3-hydroxy-3-methylglutaryl-coenzyme reductase in the hepatocyte to reduce serum total cholesterol levels by up to 30%.

Evidence: There is no evidence that the effect of statins is a drug-specific effect rather than a class effect.

Contraindications to Treatment

Contraindications include hepatic impairment, pregnancy and lactation, and porphyria.

Complications of Treatment

Statins are well tolerated, but do have occasional side effects including muscle cramps (rarely rhabdomyolysis), headaches, abdominal discomfort, and altered liver function tests.

Evidence: The Stroke Prevention by Aggressive Reduction in Choles-terol Levels (SPARCL) trial was a prospective, randomized, blinded trial of high-dose statin therapy in 4731 patients with a less than 6-month-prior stroke or TIA, but without congestive heart disease (CHD) and with normal cholesterol levels. The results at almost 5-year follow-up showed the following:

- *Recurrent fatal and nonfatal strokes were decreased in the statin-treated group (16%, p = .03), but the incidence of hemorrhagic strokes was increased in the statin-treated group (p = .02).*
- *Reduction in major coronary events (−35%, p = .003), as well as revascularization procedures in all vascular beds (coronary, carotid, and peripheral; −45%, p <.001) was observed in the statin-treated group.*
- *There was no reduction in overall mortality.*

The heart protection study was a prospective, randomized, blind trial of 20,500 people with a "high risk" of cardiovascular disease (including patients with previous TIA or stroke) and a total choles-terol of >3.5 mmol/L, randomized to either 40 mg of simvastatin or placebo for a 5-year period. The results showed the following:

- *Lowering LDL cholesterol by 1 mmol/L reduces the 5-year risk of ischemic stroke by about one fourth, with no adverse effect on*

cerebral hemorrhage. This was irrespective of age, sex, lipid levels, blood pressure, or use of other medications (including aspirin).
- *Statin therapy clearly reduces the risk of major vascular events among people with preexisting cerebrovascular disease, irrespective of the presence of coronary disease.*

Other Treatments

1. Plant stanols incorporated into food products competitively inhibit cholesterol absorption from the small bowel and so reduce serum cholesterol by 10%. This is probably additive to the effect of statins. Side effects are minimal.

   Evidence: Evidence for a direct cerebrovascular protective effect is not proven.

2. Dietary advice should always be given. At best this reduces serum cholesterol levels by 10%, but consideration of dietary intake will also manage obesity, another risk factor for stroke.

3. Fibrates lower total cholesterol concentrations less than statins, but they have larger effects on HDL and triglyceride concentrations.

4. Other lipid-lowering agents:
   a. Cholesterol transport inhibitors (ezetimibe)
   b. Cholesterol binding agents (anion-exchange resins), for example, cholestyramine, bind bile acids in the gut, stopping their reabsorption, which increases hepatic conversion of cholesterol into bile acids. The resultant increased liver cell LDL-receptor activity increases LDL-cholesterol breakdown but can aggravate hypertriglyceridemia.
   c. Omega fish oils: As there is a clear relationship between serum lipids and atherosclerosis, and reducing the serum lipid profile reduces the risk of stroke, it is probable that some of these agents are also beneficial in stroke prevention.

Bibliography

Heart Protection Study Collaborative Group. Evidence of cholesterol-lowering with simvastatin on stroke and other major vascular events in 20,536 people with cerebrovascular disease or other high risk conditions. Lancet 2004;363;757–767.

Stroke Prevention by Aggressive Reduction in Cholesterol Levels (SPARCL) Investigators. High-dose atorvastatin after stroke or transient ischemic attack. N Engl J Med 2006;355:549–559.

Chapter 10
Reducing the Risk of Stroke by Modifying Life Style

SMOKING CESSATION

Recommendations

1. All people who smoke should be encouraged to stop.
2. Those whom have suffered a cerebrovascular event should be entered into a structured smoking cessation program.

INTRODUCTION AND SIGNIFICANCE OF SMOKING

- Of all strokes 25% are due to smoking.
- Cigarette smoking independently increases the risk of stroke three-fold.
- Pipe, cigar and passive smoking are risks for atherogenesis and therefore probably stroke.
- The relative risk for stroke is the same for male and female smokers, being highest in middle age, but declining with advancing years.
- No randomized control trials have shown smoking cessation reduces stroke risk. But the risk of stroke can return to that of non-smokers within 5 years of quitting.
- From observational studies it has been estimated that in those who have had a cerebrovascular event, to cease smoking would reduce the risk of stroke (and other vascular events) from a base line annual risk of stroke of about 7% to around 5% per year, a RRR of at least 33%.

ASSESSING THE VOLUME OF SMOKING A PATIENT SELF-INFLICTS

Clinical Features
Self-reporting of smoking habits underestimates smoking status and is likely to increasingly do so as smoking becomes socially more unacceptable, and physicians forget to ask. On examination the odour of smoke and digital tar staining are often signs.

Investigations
Biochemical markers used to evaluate smoking status include measures based on thiocyanate, nicotine, cotinine and carbon monoxide levels. These measures differ widely in availability, cost and ease of administration.

TREATMENT

Method of Encouraging Smoking Cessation
A combination of counseling and medication in an ordered fashion under the guidance of a smoking cessation team is recommended.

Counseling for Smoking Cessation
Counseling, either individual or group, is more effective than using self-help material alone.

A problem-solving approach is most valuable, in which identification of highest temptation periods are managed by planning distraction strategies.

Social support in the form of encouragement, caring, and concern increases success rates. This should be from both healthcare providers (intra-treatment social support) and from family and other community members (extra-treatment social support).

If initial attempts to stop are unsuccessful, patients should encouraged to try again, stressing the short- and long-term benefits.

Medication for Smoking Cessation
Nicotine replacement therapies

These are in the form of gum, inhaler, nasal spray and patches.
They aim to relieve nicotine with drawl symptoms and urges to smoke whilst not exposing the person to carbon monoxide, tar and carcinogens in cigarette smoke.
Using nicotine replacement therapies does not appear to affect cardiovascular risks.

Side effects

  i. The patch releases nicotine slowly and therefore do not combat sudden nicotine cravings.
 ii. The main side effect is a localized rash and skin irritation which 50% experience, but only 5% actually have to stop using the product.
iii. Some patients using the 24 hour patch experience sleep disturbances.

Bupropion Bupropion is available only on prescription and should be taken only within a structured smoking cessation program.

It acts as an anti-depressant-related medication which reduces nicotine addiction centrally.

Side effects Bupropion is well tolerated.

  i. Insomnia (40%)
 ii. Dry mouth (10%)
iii. Other less common side effects include shakiness, skin irritations, headaches and dizziness. There are rare reports of serious adverse reactions including seizures and myocardial infarction.

Varenicline This is a new drug which is available only on prescription.

It acts by reducing the urge to smoke.

Treatment begins 1 week before the quit date. The dose is increased to reach 1 mg twice daily for 12 weeks. If the patient has stopped smoking at the end of the 12 weeks, another 12 weeks treatment at 1mg twice daily is considered.

Side effects Very few, but up to 30% report some nausea.
Evidence: Two randomized phase 3 comparative clinical trials report Varenicline to be superior to placebo and Bupropion.

Alternative Treatments
Therapies such as acupuncture and hypnosis are popular "alternative" ways to try to stop smoking, but no significant clinical trials support their effectiveness. The use of herbal medications such as St. John's Wart and kava kava to aid smoking cessation are also based on no clinical evidence and may even have harmful side effects or interact with other medications.

HOW WELL SUCCESSFUL IS SMOKING CESSATION AT PRESENT

In the UK the rates at which men are quitting smoking is such that today only 3 in 10 men smoke, compared with 8 in 10 at the end of the Second World War. However more women are now smoking than before. To continue to reduce smoking rates, the first phase of the *National Service Framework* on Coronary Heart Disease included a requirement for all health authorities to set up smoking cessation services; employers to have smoking policies and to help establish programmes to reduce smoking in the local communities.

22%—smoking abstinence rate after 1 year of patients *given* Varenicline

16%—smoking abstinence rate after 1 year of patients given Bupropion

8%—smoking abstinence rate after 1 year of patients given a placebo

Bibliography

Jorenby DE. Smoking cessation strategies for the 21st Century Circulation 2001;104: e51–e52

OBESITY

Recommendations

1. The dietary requirements and exercise levels of all patients should be assessed and behavioral support provided if necessary.
2. Drug and surgical intervention should be reserved for the morbidly obese, highly motivated individuals.

Overweight is a body mass index (BMI) (weight in kilograms divided by height in meters squared) of 25 to 30. A BMI between 31 and 40 is obese, and above 40 is morbidly obese. In adults over 45 years of age, two thirds are overweight or obese, and the prevalence is increasing. Obesity is more common in women in lower socioeconomic groups.

Significance

Obesity has adverse effects on many diseases, several of which are themselves cerebrovascular risk factors (Fig. 10.1). This therefore confounds the exact relationship.

For coronary disease there is a clear relationship with obesity, especially if the weight has been gained in middle age or has fluctuated substantially. Reducing weight in randomized control trials by as little as 6% leads to a reduction in blood pressure and an improvement in the diabetic and lipid profile. Extrapolated from this finding, weight reduction should reduce the risk of stroke.

Disease	Relative risk		Working days lost
	Women	Men	
Type 2 diabetes	12.7	5.2	5,960,000
Hypertension	4.2	2.6	5,160,000
Heart attack	3.2	1.5	1,230,000
Angina	1.8	1.8	2,390,000
Stroke	1.3	1.3	440,000
Working days lost are certificated absence from secondary diseases attributable to obesity			

FIGURE 10.1. Relative risk of different diseases in obese versus nonobese people (From National audit office report on Obesity).

Making the Diagnosis of Obesity

Clinical Features

1. The body mass index is the most frequently used measure of obesity. However, results are variable as it does not take into account body frame, proportion of lean mass, gender, or age.
2. Girth (waist circumference) measurements can be compared with the individual's height (the girth-height ratio [GHR]) or with the hip measurements. This is considered to be a measure of "central obesity" and is an independent and more accurate predictor of cerebrovascular and cardiovascular risk than is the BMI.
3. Longitudinal variations in body weight are probably a stronger risk factor than the BMI alone.

Treatment

Treatment is graded according to the severity of the risk of cerebrovascular disease and the actual obesity, starting with diet and exercise and then including medical intervention and reserving surgery for extreme cases.

Dietary Therapy

Patients are educated on how to adjust their diet to reduce the number of calories eaten. The aim is to reduce calorie input moderately so as to achieve a slow steady weight loss that can be maintained. This involves learning about food composition (fats, carbohydrates, and proteins), the calorie content of different foods, and how to prepare foods.

Physical Activity

Patients are encouraged to undertake moderate physical activity, building up to 30 minutes or more every day. The exercise should be aerobic (such as aerobic dancing, brisk walking, jogging, cycling, and swimming), but one that is enjoyable and can fit into their daily routine.

Behavior Therapy

Patients are taught different strategies in an attempt to change their behavior patterns to ensure weight loss. Examples of commonly used behavioral therapy strategies include the following:

1. Keeping a diet and exercise diary
2. Identifying and consciously avoiding high-risk situations
3. Setting realistic goals with regard to weight loss and exercise
4. Planning a reward system when these goals are achieved

5. Involving one's social support network (family, friends, or colleagues) or joining a support group that encourages weight loss in a positive and motivating manner

Treatment Indications. All patients following a cerebrovascular event or who have any associated risk factors should assess their weight. A combination of all three therapies is necessary, but the degree of input depends on the severity of the obesity and availability of resources.

Evidence: Dietary interventions alone do not appear to produce sustained weight loss. Behavioral interventions alone have very little effect on obesity. Diet and behavioral therapy together are more effective than diet alone. Supervised exercise classes are more effective at reducing weight than exercise education alone.

Pharmacological Interventions

Orlistat. Orlistat is a lipase inhibitor that reduces the absorption of dietary fat by up to 30%. Side effects include gastrointestinal disturbances, in particular liquid, oily stools; fecal urgency; incontinence; flatulence; and headaches and menstrual irregularities.

Sibutramine. Sibutramine acts on the central nervous system to suppress appetite, by inhibiting the reuptake of noradrenalin and serotonin. Side effects include constipation, dry mouth, and insomnia

Treatment Indications. Drug therapy is recommended for patients with either of the following:

1. BMI >30 with no obesity-related conditions
2. BMI of >27 with two or more obesity-related conditions such as type 2 diabetes, hypertension, or hypercholesterolemia

The National Institute for Clinical Excellence (NICE) guidelines suggest that drug therapy should only be considered for individuals who have lost >2.5 kg body weight in the last month by following a diet, which is controlled by an exercise regimen, and are between 18 and 75 years old. There should be continued support, usually in the form of a primary care practice nurse, to ensure that the diet and exercise regimens continue. Treatment should be stopped after 3 months if weight loss is less than 5% from the start of treatment and after 6 months if it is less than 10%. Treatment should not continue for more than a year.

Bariatric Surgical Interventions

Types of Treatment. Obesity surgery modifies the stomach and intestines to reduce the amount of food that can be eaten. Laparoscopic banded gastroplasty involves constructing a small pouch with a restricted outlet along the lesser curvature of the stomach. The outlet may be externally reinforced to prevent disruption or dilation.

Gastric bypass procedures involve constructing a proximal gastric pouch whose outlet is a Y-shaped limb of small bowel of varying lengths (Roux-en-Y gastric bypass).

Treatment Outcome. Patients are expected to lose up to 50% of their excess weight in the first 6 months and 77% of excess weight in 1 year. Patients maintain 50% of their weight loss 10 years after surgery.

Complications of Treatment. Early postoperative morbidity (10%) includes wound infections, dehiscence, leaks from staple line breakdown, stomal stenosis, and thromboembolic disorders. Later postoperative complications requiring reoperation include pouch and distal esophageal dilation, persistent vomiting, and cholecystitis. Other problems include nutrient deficiencies, particularly of vitamin B_{12}, folate, and iron.

Treatment Indications. Obesity surgery is considered for persons with either of the following:

1. BMI >40
2. BMI >35 with serious medical conditions

But the patient needs to be highly motivated and committed to making a lifestyle change after surgery. It is important that there is a full support team, including behavioral specialists and nutritionist available as part of a lifelong follow-up plan.

How well Is Obesity Managed?
Obesity has yet to be identified as a significant comorbid risk factor for cardiovascular diseases including cerebrovascular disease. The prevalence of obesity has tripled since 1980 and on present trends will continue to do so.

Bibliography
Bandolier. Obesity and health. http:/www.jr2.ox.ac.uk/bandolier/address. Effective health care: the prevention and treatment of obesity. 1997;3(2).

National Audit Office. Tackling obesity in England. Report by the Comptroller and Auditor General, HC220, session 2000–2001, February 15, 2001.http://www.nao.org.uk/publications/nao_reports/00-01/0001220.pdf.

EXERCISE AND FITNESS

Recommendations

Exercise should be encouraged in all patients at risk of a stroke. If possible this should be in the form of structured classes.

Significance

Low levels of cardiorespiratory fitness are associated with a higher risk of stroke mortality, even when adjusted for cigarette smoking, alcohol intake, body mass index, hypertension, diabetes mellitus, and parental history of coronary heart disease. However, there are no studies to show that increasing exercise and thus cardiorespiratory fitness reduces the risk of stroke. But this assertion is based on the following findings:

1. Exercise effectively reduces events in other vascular beds, such that moderate to high levels of physical activity reduce the relative risk of coronary events by 40%, and exercise improves peripheral vascular disease symptoms.
2. Exercise reduces several cerebrovascular risk factors. Aerobic exercise has been shown to do the following:
   a. Lower the patient's blood pressure (particularly in hypertensive patients)
   b. Improve the patient's lipid profile (i.e., promote a decrease in levels of total blood cholesterol, serum triglycerides, and LDL cholesterol, and increase HDL cholesterol
   c. Enhance glucose regulation
   d. Promote a decrease in body weight and fat stores

Exercise also improves the quality of life by increasing bone density; improving strength, stamina, coordination, balance, and flexibility; as well as improving one's sense of well-being and reducing stress.

Assessing the Fitness of a Patient

Clinical Features

Fitness levels depend on the patient's previous exercise history, age, body type, smoking history, and medical history. A good indication of current fitness is the resting heart rate and the speed with which the heart rate returns to this level after moderate exercise.

Investigations

There are several tests that can be undertaken to determine general fitness. These need to be adapted to the individual patient who has had a cerebrovascular event. They aim to assess cardiorespiratory endurance or stamina with walking, running, cycling, or step tests, and muscle strength and endurance by assessing the duration for which a muscle contraction can be held.

Treatment

Preexercise Evaluation. Before starting the exercise program, the individual is fully assessed. This should involve a complete medical history and physical examination, as well as graded exercise testing with electrocardiogram (ECG) monitoring. It is wise to undertake this assessment in a rehabilitation unit as the tests will have to be adapted to the abilities of the stroke patient.

Exercise Programs. Each exercise session should begin with a warm up, followed by stretching, the actual aerobic exercise, and then a cool down and stretch. The exercise-programming recommendations for stroke survivors by the American Heart Association is summarized in Fig. 10.2. Treadmill walking is recommended as the mainstay of the aerobic exercise, but resistance, flexibility, and neuromuscular training are also included.

Initially exercising is for a short time (e.g., 10 minutes) on nonconsecutive days (e.g., 3 days a week) with a small amount of effort. Gradually the frequency and duration of the aerobic exercise is increased before increasing the intensity. Although it is important to have a structured exercise class, as this produces the best results, it is important for patients to take possession of the activity and incorporate it into their daily activities.

Involve the patient's social support network (family, friends or colleagues) or suggest that the patient join a support group that encourages weight loss in a positive and motivating manner.

Complications of Treatment

The major complication is musculoskeletal injuries.

How Successfully Is Exercise Encouraged?

Sixty percent of people are not active enough to benefit their health, especially in the older age groups. This number has increased over the last 25 years.

Mode of Exercise	Goals	Intensity/Frequency/Duration
Aerobic • Large-muscle activities (eg, walking, treadmill, stationary cycle, combined arm-leg ergometry, arm ergometry, seated stepper)	• Increase independence in ADLs • Increase walking speed/efficiency • Improve tolerance for prolonged physical activity • Reduce cardiovascular disease risks	• 40%–70% peak oxygen uptake; 40%–70% heart rate reserve; 50%–80% maximal heart rate; RPE 11–14 (6–20 scale) • 3–7 d/wk • 20–60 min/session (or multiple 10-min sessions)
Strength • Circuit training • Weight machines • Free weights • Isometric exercise	• Increase independence in ADLs	• 1–3 sets of 10–15 repetitions of 8–10 exercises involving the major muscle groups • 2–3 d/wk
Flexibility • Stretching	• Increase ROM of involved extremities • Prevent contractures	• 2–3 d/wk (before or after aerobic or strength training) • Hold each stretch for 10–30 seconds
Neuromuscular • Coordination and balance activities	• Improve level of safety during ADLs	• 2–3 d/wk (consider performing on same day as strength activities)

ADLs indicates activities of daily living; RPE, rating of perceived exertion; and ROM, range of motion.

Recommended intensity, frequency, and duration of exercise depend on each individual patient's level of fitness. Intermittent training sessions may be indicated during the initial weeks of rehabilitation.

FIGURE 10.2. Exercise Programming Recommendations for Stroke Survivors (Gordon et al 2004).

Bibliography

Gordon NF, et al. Physical activity and exercise recommendations for stroke survivors. Circulation 2004;109:2031–2041. http://circ.ahajournals.org/cgi/content/full/109/16/2031.

Wendel-Vos GCW, Schuit AJ, Feskens EJM, et al. Physical activity and stroke. A meta-analysis of observational data. Int J Epidemiol 2004;33(4):787–798.

DIET MODIFICATION

Diet modulation affects obesity and the level of fitness. Specific dietary modifications affect other cerebrovascular risk factors including hyperhomocystinemia, blood pressure, and hyperlipidemia.

Diet Modification to Affect Hyperhomocystinemia

> **Recommendations**
>
> Consider homocystine-lowering vitamins (folic acid, vitamin B_{12}, and probably vitamin B_6) only in patients with proven high homocystine levels who have suffered a cerebrovascular event, as it may have an effect on cardiovascular morbidity.

Homocysteine is a sulfur-containing amino acid formed from methionine, which itself is derived from dietary proteins. Homocysteine is metabolibed by either remethylation, which requires vitamin B_{12} and folic acid, or by a trans-sulfuration pathway, which requires vitamin B_6. Circulating homocysteine levels are therefore a product of methionine intake and homocystien metabolism, which may be folate or vitamin B dependent.

In patients with raised homocystein levels, taking a combination of folic acid, vitamin B_{12}, and possibly vitamin B_6 reduces these levels by up to 30%.

Significance

Good laboratory evidence suggests that free circulating homocysteine stimulates atherosclerotic vessel wall changes. Clinically, although systemic reviews of observational studies have shown a higher incidence of raised plasma homocystine levels in patients with atherosclerotic diseases including cerebrovascular disease, prospective cohort studies have failed to find an association, and randomized control trials have failed to show that lowering raised homocystine levels reduces the risk of cerebrovascular events.

Evidence: The VITAmins TO Prevent Stroke (VITATOPS) study randomized 285 patients with cerebrovascular events to receive "vitamins" including folate and showed that although baseline homocysteine levels fell, this was not a significant reduction and had no effect on the subsequent stroke rate.

The Vitamin Intervention for Stroke Prevention (VISP) trial randomized 3680 patients to homocystine-lowering vitamins and showed a moderate fall in total homocysteine after stroke had no effect on vascular outcomes.

Making the Diagnosis of Hyperhomocystinemia
Homocysteine is measured from a nonfasting blood sample. A normal level is <12 µmol/L.

Treatment Indications

Primary Prevention
The American Heart Association does not feel that there is sufficient evidence for reducing homocysteine levels as a prevention of cardiovascular disease and stroke that warrants recommending the widespread use of folic acid and B vitamin supplements. However, it does advise a healthy, balanced diet that includes at least five servings of fruits and vegetables a day to obtain adequate levels of folic acid (400 µg/day) and vitamin B_6.

Secondary Prevention
Patients who have suffered a cerebrovascular event and have homocysteine levels >12.5 µmol/L could be considered for treatment with a combination of folic acid, vitamin B_{12}, and vitamin B_6. In patients with levels lower than this, advice should be as for primary prevention.

Complications of Treatment
There are very few side effects and most are minor gastrointestinal symptoms such as anorexia, nausea, flatulence, and abdominal distention.

Bibliography
Christen WG, Ajani UA, Glynn RJ, Hennekens CH. Blood levels of homocysteine and increased risk of cardiovascular disease: causal or casual? Arch Intern Med 2000;160:422–434.

Eilelboom JW, Lonn E, Genest J, et al. Homocysteine and cardiovascular disease: a critical review of the epidemiologic evidence. Ann Intern Med 1999;131:363–375.

Hankey GJ, Eikelboom JW, Loh K, et al. Sustained homocysteine-lowering effect over time of folic acid-based multivitamin therapy in stroke patients despite increasing folate status in the population. Cerebrovasc Dis 2005;19(2):110–116. Epub 2004 December 17.

Homocysteine Lowering Trialists' Collaboration. Lowering blood homocysteine with folic acid based supplements: meta-analysis of randomized trials. Br Med J 1998;316:894–898.

Toole JF, Malinow MR, Chambless LE, et al. Lowering homocysteine in patients with ischemic stroke to prevent recurrent stroke, myocardial infarction, and death: the Vitamin Intervention for Stroke Prevention (VISP) randomized controlled trial. JAMA 2004;291(5): 565–575.

DIET MODIFICATION TO AFFECT BLOOD PRESSURE

Salt Restriction

Systemic reviews of randomized trials suggests that salt restriction leads to modest reductions in blood pressure, having a greater benefit in older people. A mean reduction of sodium intake by 6.7 g per day for 28 days leads to a 3.8 mm Hg reduction in systolic blood pressure.

Potassium and fish oil supplements do reduce blood pressure a little (about 5 mm Hg systolic), but in themselves have not demonstrated a reduced risk of stroke.

Antioxidant supplements have not been shown to be of any benefit and may be harmful in the case of beta-carotene.

DIET MODIFICATION TO AFFECT SERUM LIPID LEVELS

The use of plant stanols, dietary restrictions, and fish oils to lower plasma cholesterol levels has been discussed earlier.

ALCOHOL AS A RISK FOR STROKE

Heavy alcohol consumption, including binge drinking, is an independent and causal factor for stroke, although this is more likely to be a hemorrhagic than an ischemic stroke.

However, it is likely that moderate alcohol consumption may have a cerebrovascular protective effect.

Coffee consumption is not associated with an increased risk of stroke

Chapter 11
Identifying Other Atherosclerotic Diseases

Atherosclerosis affects several vascular beds. The presence of disease in one bed increases the likelihood of disease in another. It is necessary to assess the increased risk of stroke in patients who suffer disease in another vascular bed. This includes peripheral vascular disease, ischemic heart disease, and renal artery disease.

PATIENTS AT AN INCREASED RISK OF STROKE DUE TO ASSOCIATED PERIPHERAL VASCULAR DISEASE

Recommendations

1. Determine a cerebrovascular history in patients with peripheral vascular disease.
2. Consider duplex scanning the carotid arteries of patients with peripheral vascular disease.

Peripheral arterial occlusive vascular disease affects 10% of the population over the age of 60 years. It is often asymptomatic, and in most cases, when symptomatic, presents as intermittent claudication with calf and other leg muscles painfully cramping only on exercise. The symptoms are relieved within a moment or two once exercise has stopped. In 10% of cases the disease progresses to a critical stage where there is persistent ischemic foot pain or gangrene and ulceration and the limb is threatened.

Significance

Patients with peripheral vascular disease, as determined by a reduced ankle-brachial pressure index (ABPI), are at an increased risk of stroke, even when the peripheral vascular disease is asymptomatic.

The prevalence of stroke in claudicant patients is 36% versus 11% in a controlled population; 20% of claudicant patients die from a stroke. The exact etiology of the stroke in claudicant patients is not known, but almost 30% are lacunar infarct strokes (and probably not due to macroembolization), and 12% of patients with claudication who have no cerebrovascular symptoms have an associated >70% carotid artery bifurcation stenosis. The percentage of peripheral vascular disease patients with asymptomatic carotid artery stenoses of >70% may reach as high as 30% in those with critical limb ischemia.

The prevalence of claudication among stroke patients is 10%, and although they have a similar mortality and functional resolution to nonclaudicant patients, claudication is an independent risk factor for death within 5 years of a stroke.

Making the Diagnosis of Peripheral Vascular Disease
The diagnosis of peripheral vascular disease is made primarily on clinical features. The diagnosis and severity of the disease is confirmed by the ABPI. If it is less than 0.8, the patient is likely to have claudication, and if below 0.3, the patient is likely to be suffering critical limb ischemia. Investigations such as duplex ultrasound scanning and computed tomography (CT) angiography are only undertaken if peripheral vascular intervention is considered.

Treatment Indications
Peripheral vascular disease management is twofold:

1. Controlling cardiovascular risk factors such as stopping smoking, taking antiplatelet medication, and controlling hypertension, diabetes, and hypercholesterolemia, all of which are important for primary cerebrovascular disease prevention.
2. With regard to the peripheral vascular disease itself, in claudicant patients management focuses on structured exercise classes, and this is also an important part of primary cerebrovascular disease management.

The incidence of asymptomatic carotid artery stenoses is higher in those with peripheral vascular disease, and some advocate a screening carotid artery duplex in such patients. This has not been subjected to any significant clinical trials and is not universally undertaken.

PATIENTS AT AN INCREASED RISK OF STROKE DUE TO ASSOCIATED AORTIC ANEURYSM

Silent cerebrovascular infarcts are higher in patients with infrarenal abdominal aortic aneurysms. There is no direct cause and effect except that several of the risk factors associated with aortic aneurysms are also associated risks for stroke, in particular smoking and hypertension.

PATIENTS AT AN INCREASED RISK OF STROKE DUE TO ASSOCIATED RENAL INSUFFICIENCY

Recommendations

Control all cerebrovascular risk factors.

Chronic renal failure affects 2 of 1000 people. Diabetes and hypertension are the two commonest causes and account for two thirds of cases.

Significance

A raised serum creatinine level, even within the normal range, is associated with an increased risk of stroke, after adjustment for confounding factors, such as hypertension. This risk is greater in men with no evidence of preexisting ischemic heart disease.

Silent infarcts are found more often in people with severe renal failure than in those with no renal failure.

The mortality following a stroke in patients with impaired renal function is higher than in those without (even after adjustment for confounder factors such as age, neurological score, ischemic heart disease,hypertension, smoking, and diuretic use).

Cardiovascular disease is the major cause of death among patients with end-stage renal disease. In such patients cardiovascular mortality is 30-fold greater than among the general population.

No study has demonstrated that the incidence of stroke is reduced by modifying the rate of renal failure deterioration. However, as renal disease is often associated with several cardiovascular risk factors such as diabetes and hypertension and controlling these in renal failure patients reduces the incidence of cardiac events, it is probably also the case for stroke.

Making the Diagnosis of Renal Failure

Clinical Features
Initial symptoms include unintentional weight loss, nausea, vomiting, generally malaise, frequent hiccups, and generalized pruritus.

Investigations
Blood chemistry shows a worsening serum creatinine and urea levels, a raised potassium, with a metabolic acidosis.

Treatment
Treatment aims to control symptoms, minimize complications, and slow disease progression. This often involves fluid intake and dietary protein, salt, potassium, and phosphorus restrictions. All cardiovascular risk factors must be controlled.

Chapter 12
Managing Lacunar Infarcts

> **Recommendations**
>
> 1. Patients with lacunar infarcts require full cerebrovascular assessment, including, assessment of extracerebral sources of emboli.
> 2. All cerebrovascular risk factors need to be aggressively managed.

A lacunar infarct is a small brain infarct due to occlusion of a penetrating branch of a large cerebral artery, occurring mainly in the basal ganglia. It should not be considered as a separate entity, as it is associated with several cerebrovascular risk factors that can be controlled.

SIGNIFICANCE

Twenty percent of ischemic cerebrovascular events are associated with lacunar infarcts. Patients with lacunar infarcts are more likely to improve and generally have a better prognosis than other causes of stroke (30-day mortality <5%). The recurrence rate following a lacunar stroke over several years is 10%. Only a minority of recurrent strokes have a lacunar etiology.

Lacunar infarcts are caused by the following:

1. Intrinsic microatheromatous disease of the penetrating arteries (also called lipohyalinosis) associated in particular with hypertension.
2. Embolic occlusion of penetrating vessels (including cardioemboli in 12% of cases compared to 25% of causes in nonlacunar infarcts).
3. Unusual causes include polycythemia, cholesterol emboli, and vasculitis.

The associated risk factors for developing lacunar infarcts are aging, hypertension, diabetes mellitus, hyperlipidemia, and smoking.

MAKING THE DIAGNOSIS OF LACUNAR INFARCTS

Clinical Features
Four neurological syndromes have been described to suggest a lacunar infarct: pure motor hemiparesis (50% of lacunar cases), pure hemisensory loss (5%), hemisensorimotor loss (35%), and ataxic hemiparesis (10%). For each there is no visual field defect, no other cortical defect such as speech, no impairment of consciousness, and no brainstem symptoms.

The lacunar syndromes are not pathognomonic of a lacunar infarct, as larger strokes and embolic strokes can also manifest clinically as lacunar syndromes.

Investigations
The diagnosis of lacunar infarcts is made on the basis of brain imaging, in particular computed tomography (CT) and magnetic resonance imaging (MRI). On CT they appear as small punctate hypodense foci in the basal ganglia and deep white matter. On MRI they are better seen on T2-weighted images where they appear as rounded or slit-like hyperintense foci.

TREATMENT
Hypertension, needs to be treated aggressively. As lacunar infarcts are often to be associated with an extracranial source of emboli which need to be identified and controlled. Other cerebrovascular risks factors such as diabetes and smoking need to be managed.

HOW WELL ARE LACUNAR INFARCTS RISK FACTORS BEING MANAGED?
The frequency of lacunae in autopsy studies has fallen from 11% in the 1950s to 8% in the 1970s, which may be due to more extensive antihypertension management.

Part IV
Reducing the Risk of Stroke by Reducing Procoagulant (Thrombotic) Risk Factors

Chapter 13
Managing Procoagulant Thrombotic States

A procoagulant/thrombotic state results from either a disturbance in hemostasis or an alteration in the viscosity of the blood components (Table. 13.1). Both potentially increase the risk of ischemic stroke.

MANAGING THROMBOPHILIA (DISTURBANCES IN COAGULATION/ANTICOAGULATION CASCADE)

> **Recommendations**
>
> Consider lifelong anticoagulation only in patients in whom no other cause of stoke is established, or who are young.

In thrombophilic disorders there is an increased tendency to form intravascular venous or arterial thrombosis, with laboratory evidence of abnormal hemostasis. Although factor V Leiden occurs in 6% of the normal population (and in 20% of patients with deep venous thrombosis [DVT], and 60% with recurrent DVT), other disorders are much rarer, with protein C and S and antithrombin III deficiencies having a prevalence of 0.05% in the general population.

Significance
Known hematologic abnormalities account for 4% of all strokes. This proportion is higher in younger people.

Of the inherited thrombophilias, factor V Leiden and the prothrombin 20210 mutation are statistically only associated with stroke in children and adults under age 40. This risk of

TABLE 13.1. Hematological disorders associated with ischemic stroke (common causes of a prothrombotic state)

I. Thrombophilia disorders

    1. Hereditary deficiencies of natural coagulant inhibitors
       a. Antithrombin III
       b. Protein C
       c. Protein S
    2. Single point mutations in coagulation molecules
       a. Factor V Leiden (activated protein C resistance)
       b. Factor II; 20210G/A
    3. Hereditary disorders of fibrinolysisplasminogen deficiency
    4. Antiphospholipid syndrome

II. Myeloproliferative disorders

    1. Essential thrombocythemia
    2. Polycythemia rubra vera

III. Other causes

    1. Platelet disorders
       a. Thrombotic thrombocytopenic purpura
       b. Heparin-induced thrombocytopenia
    2. Erythrocyte disorders
       a. Sickle cell disease
    3. Paraproteinemias
    4. Nephritic syndrome
    5. Cancer including intravascular lymphoma and leukemia
    6. Pregnancy and the oral contraceptive pill

stroke is substantially increased by concomitant exposure to oral contraceptives.

Of the acquired thrombophilias, the antiphospholipid antibody syndrome is present in 10% of acute ischemic stroke. This percentage is higher in younger patients.

Antithrombin III deficiency and protein C and protein S deficiencies are associated with venous thrombosis, and there is no strong evidence to support an association with ischemic stroke.

Usually the hematological disorder is one of several factors predisposing to thrombus formation, and it is difficult to confidently assert that the disorder is the main cause of an ischemic stroke.

Making the Diagnosis of a Thrombophilia

Clinical Features
A thrombophilia should be suspected in ischemic stroke patients who are <50 years with the following findings:

1. No obvious cause of stroke
2. A history of multiple unexplained strokes
3. A prior history of venous thrombosis
4. Family history of thrombosis
5. Abnormalities on routine screening coagulation tests

Antiphospholipid syndrome is suspected in patients with a history of multiple miscarriages, dementia, optic neuropathy, or thrombocytopenia.

Investigations
Thrombophilia screening assays are becoming increasingly accurate. Most hematology units run selected tests and should be consulted.

Treatment
The exact risk of a recurrent cerebrovascular event in a patient with an inherited thrombophilia is not clear. In general, the association is ignored if other strong risk factors for stroke are identified, but in patients in whom no other cause is established, or who are young, lifelong anticoagulation should be considered.

Complications of Treatment
For patients with protein C or S deficiency, treatment with heparin at the initiation of warfarin therapy reduces the risk of skin necrosis.

MANAGING SICKLE CELL DISEASE

Recommendations

1. Children with sickle cell disease should have transcranial Doppler monitoring.
2. If the peak systolic velocity is raised, or they have a stroke they should receive repeated blood transfusions.

Sickle cell disease and its variants are genetic disorders of hemoglobins that alter the oxygen carrying capacity and shape of the erythrocyte, and present with chronic hemolytic anemia and vaso-occlusive crises including stroke. The sickle gene is present in approximately 8% of black Americans but is present in as many as 30% in some areas of Africa.

Significance
Children with sickle cell disease are 300 times as likely to suffer a stroke, compared to children without the disease; 10% will develop stroke by adulthood, but 20% will have infarcts on brain magnetic resonance imaging scans.

Approximately two thirds of children who have a stroke will have a recurrent stroke. Most strokes are infarcts in the distribution of the internal carotid artery or the middle or anterior cerebral arteries. The peak incidence is between 4 and 6 years of age

Clinical Features
Sickle cell disease is present mostly in blacks. It also is found, with much less frequency, in eastern Mediterranean and Middle East populations. It usually presents with a sickle crisis in which there is severe deep pain in the extremities, involving long bones, the abdomen, and sometimes the face. The pain may be accompanied by fever, malaise, and leukocytosis.

Investigations
1. Full blood count and film will identify sickled erythrocytes and anemia. The reticulocyte count will confirm the briskness of the marrow response to the anemia.
2. Hemoglobin electrophoresis establishes the diagnosis by demonstrating a single band of Hb S (in Hb SS) or Hb S with mutant hemoglobin in compound heterozygotes.
3. Certain genetic mutations appear to carry a higher likelihood of stroke in sickle cell sufferers. Future identification of these subgroups may help in targeting treatment.
4. Transcranial Doppler screening of the middle cerebral artery should be undertaken in all children with sickle cell disease. Those with increased velocities (indicating a possible stenosis) should be considered for chronic transfusion therapy, maintaining the level of Hb S at 30% or less.

Treatment

Repeated blood transfusions maintaining the level of Hb S at 30% or less reduces the risk of stroke. There is a suggestion that after 30 transfusions the incidence of stroke may be more permanently abated.

Evidence: The Stroke Prevention Trial in Sickle Cell Anemia (STOP) (I and II) trials showed that children at highest risk of experiencing a first stroke were 10 times more likely to have a stroke if untreated when compared to high-risk children treated with chronic blood transfusion therapy. High-risk children were identified using transcranial Doppler ultrasound

Complications of Treatment

Risks of transfusion include infection, allosensitization, and iron overload.

Bibliography

Adams RJ. Lessons from the Stroke Prevention Trial in Sickle Cell Anemia (STOP) study. J Child Neurol 2000;15(5):344–349.

MANAGING MYELOPROLIFERATIVE DISORDERS

Myeloproliferative disorders are neoplastic (clonal) disorders of hemopoietic stem cells, which result in overproduction of all cell lines, with usually one line in particular. The alteration in blood constituents can result in cerebrovascular events, contributing to 1% of ischemic strokes.

The myeloproliferative disorders include the following:

1. Essential (primary) thrombocythemia
2. Polycythemia (rubra) vera
3. Myelofibrosis (with myeloid metaplasia), agnogenic myeloid metaplasia

Essential (Primary) Thrombocythemia

Essential thrombocythemia is a neoplastic stem cell disorder in which large numbers of abnormal platelets are produced.Abnormal platelets aggregate, causing thrombosis and occasionally bleeding. It is a rare disease with an incidence of 1.5/100,000. Essential thrombocythemia is distinguished from secondary thrombocythemia, which can occur in response to inflammation, acute bleeding, iron deficiency, splenectomy, and infection.

Significance
Of all ischemic strokes, 0.5% are attributed to essential thrombocythemia; 12.5% of all patients with essential thrombocythemia have an ischemic stroke.

Clinical Features
1. Erythromelalgia
2. Vascular occlusive disorders such as stroke, peripheral vascular disease, and ischemic heart disease
3. Bleeding (easy bruising and petechiae, unusually heavy or prolonged bleeding, nose or gum bleeding)

In some cases there are no clinical features.

Laboratory Findings
1. A platelet count above 600×10^9/L
2. A positive endogenous megakaryocyte or erythroid colony growth from blood

Treatment
1. Platelet reduction treatment using hydroxyurea, a nonalkylating agent, in patients with essential thrombocythemia and high risk of thrombosis (>60 years and a previous thrombotic event)
2. Antiplatelet agents (aspirin)

Polycythemia Rubra Vera
Polycythemia rubra vera is a neoplastic (clonal) stem cell disorder, which leads to excessive production of all myeloid cell lines, but predominantly red cells. The increase in whole blood viscosity causes vascular occlusion and ischemia stroke, compounded by the increase in platelets.

Significance
A rare disease with an incidence of 2.8/100,000. A cerebrovascular event may precede the diagnosis in 35% of patients with polycythemia rubra vera.

Clinical Features
There are no symptoms at early stages. In later stages, symptoms can include the following:

1. Headaches
2. Pruritus
3. Fullness in the upper abdomen (enlarged liver and spleen)
4. Bleeding tendency

INVESTIGATIONS

1. Full blood count, which shows raised hematocrit as well as raised platelets and white blood cells.
2. Blood samples, which may also show elevated erythrocyte sedimentation rate (ESR), cholesterol, and uric acid.
3. Bone marrow biopsy, which makes the diagnosis.

Treatment

1. Phlebotomy to obtain a hematocrit >0.45
2. Low-dose aspirin (if already had a stroke), 75 mg/day
3. Hydroxyurea if necessary
4. Do not treat with iron

Table 13.1 lists the hematological disorders associated with ischemic stroke

Part V
Reducing the Risk of Stroke from Other Causes

Chapter 14
Managing Central Nervous System Vasculitis

> **Recommendations**
>
> All patients who have suffered a cerebrovascular event should have the erythrocyte sedimentation rate (ESR) measured.

Vasculitis (angiitis, arteritis) is a general category of approximately 20 disorders that involve inflammation of blood vessels, which have varied etiologies and pathologies. When the vasculitis involves the central nervous system vessels it is one of the following types:

1. Primary (primary angiitis of the central nervous system [PACNS]) when there is no other condition to cause the blood vessels damage
2. Secondary, as part of a systemic diseases and vasculitides such as systemic lupus erythematosus (SLE), Sjgren's syndrome, Wegener's granulomatosis, polyarteritis nodosa, and temporal arteritis.

Secondary CNS vasculitis can also be caused by a drug reaction (e.g., amphetamines, cocaine). Secondary causes are more common than are primary causes. Temporal arteritis is the most common form of vasculitis that occurs in adults usually over the age of 50 years. The mechanism of stroke varies, but it is usually necrotizing vasculitis, hypercoagulable state, or embolism from the heart or other arteries.

SIGNIFICANCE
Seven percent of cases of temporal arteritis have transient ischemic attacks (TIAs) or stroke.

CLINICAL FEATURES

1. Neurological symptoms of CNS vasculitis
   a. Stroke due to abrupt occlusion of vessels
   b. TIAs
   c. Amaurosis fugax
   d. Waxing and waning of multiple symptoms over many months, including weakness of the arms and legs when the spinal cord is involved
2. Severe headache unresponsive to usual therapy
3. Less specific symptoms
   a. Profound loss of memory and concentration (i.e., dementia),
   b. An altered level of consciousness
   c. Problems with bowel or bladder function

INVESTIGATIONS

Markers of inflammation such as a raised ESR are combined with clinical features to suggest a vasculitis, but no simple tests can secure the diagnosis of CNS vasculitis.

1. Cerebral spinal fluid analysis excludes other diagnoses.
2. CT and MRI scans are unable to distinguish CNS vasculitis from other forms of neurologic disease.
3. Cerebral arteriography identifies nonspecific changes that cannot be distinguished from atherosclerosis vessel changes. Any cerebral vessel spasm during the procedure can mimic the changes seen in CNS vasculitis.
4. Biopsy
   a. Brain biopsy is the most direct means of making the diagnosis of CNS vasculitis, and should be reserved for cases in which a secondary cause has been excluded.
   b. Temporal artery biopsy should be taken from the clinically affected side and is positive in 70% of patients with temporal arteritis (20% with polymyalgia rheumatica).

TREATMENT

Primary Prevention

If temporal arteritis is suspected (jaw claudication, tenderness over temporal arteries, raised ESR, and positive biopsy), blindness and stroke can be prevented by prescribing high-dose steroids.

Primary CNS vasculitis, proven by biopsy, requires aggressive high-dose steroid and cyclophosphamide for 6 to 12 months, and requires meticulous follow-up to assess benefit and avoid side effects.

Secondary CNS vasculitis requires treatment of the underlying cause, which often involves steroid use.

Chapter 15
Managing Stroke in Human Immunodeficiency Virus–Infected Patients

Stroke affects 0.5% to 7% of acquired immune deficiency syndrome (AIDS) patients, but is found in 20% of autopsy studies (i.e., most are silent); 99% of strokes in AIDS are occlusive.

Causes specific to HIV include the following:

1. Hypertension, secondary to HIV nephropathy
2. Coagulopathies
3. Mycotic aneurysms
4. Specific forms of heart disease (infectious myocarditis lymphocytic endocarditis)
5. Cerebral vasculitis

INVESTIGATIONS
Non-HIV causes for stroke need to be excluded.

TREATMENT
Management of cerebrovascular disease in HIV-positive patients depends on the underlying cause and is not specific to HIV. However, it can be complicated by the involvement of several different physicians and multiple drug regimens that may interact.

Chapter 16
Thyroid Diseases and Stroke

> **Recommendations**
>
> A clinical and biochemical thyroid disease screen should be undertaken in all cerebrovascular patients

---

Thyroid disease is associated with an increased risk of stroke, because the disease precipitates other cerebrovascular risks.

CAUSES OF STROKE IN HYPERTHYROIDISM

Thyrotoxicosis or hyperthyroidism describes the appearance of patients in which there is an excessive amount of circulating thyroid hormone, irrespective of the origin.

Subclinical hyperthyroidism is defined as a low-serum thyroid-stimulating hormone (TSH) concentration, when serum-free thyroxine and free triiodothyronine concentrations are normal.

ATRIAL FIBRILLATION (AF) AND CARDIOEMBOLIC STROKE

Atrial fibrillation occurs in 15% of patients with hyperthyroidism. The prevalence increases with age to over 25% of hyperthyroid patients over the age of 60.

The prevalence of hyperthyroidism in patients with atrial fibrillation is 4%.

It is more common in men than women.

1. *Treatment.* Treating the hyperthyroidism to obtain a euthyroid state often results in spontaneous reversion to sinus rhythm within 6 weeks. If sinus rhythm has not occurred within 4 months of reaching a euthyroid state, it is unlikely to occur.

2. *Anticoagulation*. There is controversy over anticoagulation during the hyperthyroid state as there is believed to be an increased likelihood of bleeding. In general, anticoagulation is considered appropriate. Hyperthyroid patients are often more sensitive to warfarin

In a euthyroid-treated state, the atrial fibrillation should be treated with anticoagulation.

HYPERCOAGULABLE STATES
An association between hyperthyroidism and antiphospholipid syndrome has been suggested as the aetiology for an increased incidence of central vein thrombosis-caused stroke. This is a very rare diagnosis, and the relationship is tenuous

GIANT CELL ARTERITIS
Graves disease may be associated with Giant Cell arteritis. The prevalence of hyperthyroidism is 6 times higher in patients with Giant Cell arteritis than in controls.

CAUSES OF STROKE IN HYPOTHYROIDSIM
• Coronary artery atherosclerosis is twice as common in patients with hypothyroidism. Obtaining a eurthyroid state probably protects against progression.
• It has not been shown that hypothyroidism has a direct effect on stroke, but it is presumed so by extrapolation from coronary data.
• Hypothroidism has a strong influence on several atherosclerotic risk factors. It is associated with

   i. elevated low-density lipoprotein (LDL) cholesterol levels,
   ii. hypertension,
   iii. hyper-homocysteinemia,
   iv. synergistic effect between smoking and hypothyroidism. Smokers with hypothyroidism have higher serum cholesterol levels,
   v. coagulation profile can be altered.

Bibliography
A. Squizzato, et al. Thyroid Diseases and Cerebrovascular Disease *Stroke*. 2005;36:2302.

Part VI

Prevention of Other
Cardiovascular Events
in Cerebrovascular Patients

Chapter 17
Management of Silent Myocardial Ischemia in Stroke Patients

Recommendations

1. Assess risk of coronary heart disease in all stroke patients.
2. Treat stroke patients with a high risk of coronary heart disease.

Atherosclerosis affects several vascular beds. The presence of disease in one increases the likelihood of disease in another. Although most patients who suffer a stroke will die from a cerebrovascular event, 20% will die for other cardiovascular causes (Fig. 17.1). It is therefore important to identify and minimize the risks in all vascular beds.

SIGNIFICANCE

Patients who have had a cerebrovascular event have a 30% prevalence of silent coronary heart disease (i.e., clinically asymptomatic with normal resting electrocardiogram [ECG] but ischemic abnormalities on stress testing). This is higher if there is associated carotid artery stenosis (50%) and lower in lacunar infarcts (20%).

The prevalence of overt coronary heart disease, as manifested by a history of myocardial infarction, coronary artery bypass surgery, or current angina, in stroke patients is 25%. However, stroke patients are at a low increased risk for cardiac-related death in the short and intermediate term:

1. Three percent of patients with acute ischemic stroke have fatal cardiac-related events within 90 days after stroke.

2. The risk of cardiac-related events after stroke in the intermediate term (3 to 24 months) in patients being treated with
antiplatelet agents who do not have an established history of
cardiovascular disease is also low, possibly in the range of 2%
per year.

This is not the case in the long term, where stroke patients are at
a high risk of death from coronary heart disease, being at least
twofold that of age-matched controls and accounts for a third of
the late mortality from stroke. Mortality is higher in patients with
large-artery strokes (carotid artery stenoses) than in patients with
small-artery/lacunar stroke.

   With regard to coronary heart disease and carotid endarterectomy surgical risks, large retrospective analyses have demonstrated a significant association between a preoperative coronary
heart disease history and surgical risk, including operative
mortality and early and late postoperative cardiac morbidity.

IDENTIFYING STROKE PATIENTS AT RISK OF SILENT MYOCARDIAL ISCHEMIA

The American Heart Association recommends that the risk of
coronary heart disease be assessed in stroke patients in the
following ways:

1. Comprehensive cardiovascular risk scoring systems: Such
   scoring systems are based on the patient's history and workup
   and compared with data obtained from, for example, the
   Framingham Study and the Global Risk Assessment Scoring.
2. Noninvasive coronary heart provocation tests such as exercise
   ECG, nuclear myocardial perfusion imaging, and stress
   echocardiography, especially in those at high risk.

TREATMENT OF SILENT MYOCARDIAL ISCHEMIA IN CEREBROVASCULAR PATIENTS

1. Risk factor modification, which is same as that recommended
   for cerebrovascular disease.
2. Invasive revascularization intervention (coronary bypass
   surgery, angioplasty) should be considered.

Cerebrovascular patients with silent myocardial ischemia have a
poor prognosis, similar to those with symptomatic myocardial
ischemia, which is worse than that of an age- and sex-matched
population without silent ischemia. Intervention favorably alters
prognosis.

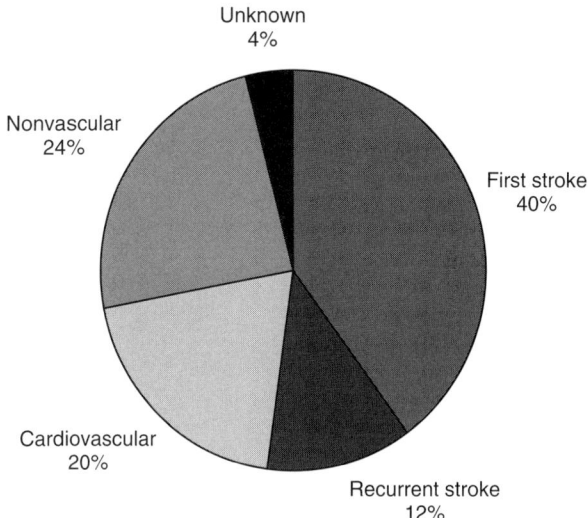

FIGURE 17.1. Cause of death over 5 years following a cerebrovascular event. (From data of 370 patients of which 58% had died at 5 years, from Hankey GJ, Jamrozik K, Broadhurst RJ, et al. Five-year survival after first-ever stroke and related prognostic factors in the Perth Community Stroke Study. Stroke 2000;31(9):2080-2086).

Bibliography

Adams RJ, Chimowitz MI, Alpert JS, et al., Stroke Council and the Council on Clinical Cardiology of the American Heart Association, American Stroke Association. Coronary risk evaluation in patients with transient ischemic attack and ischemic stroke: a scientific statement for healthcare professionals from the Stroke Council and the Council on Clinical Cardiology of the American Heart Association/American Stroke Association. Circulation 2003;108(10):1278–1290.

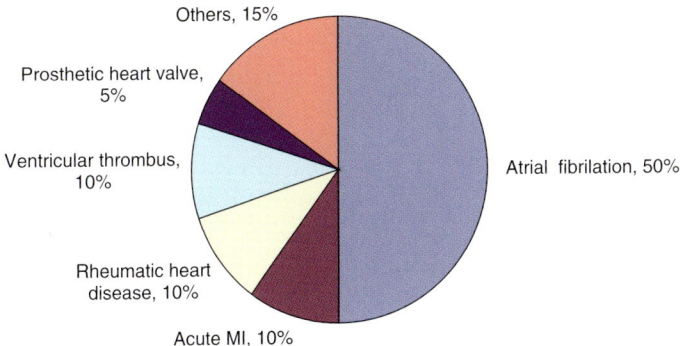

COLOR PLATE 1. Sources of cardioembolic stroke. [*See* page 25].

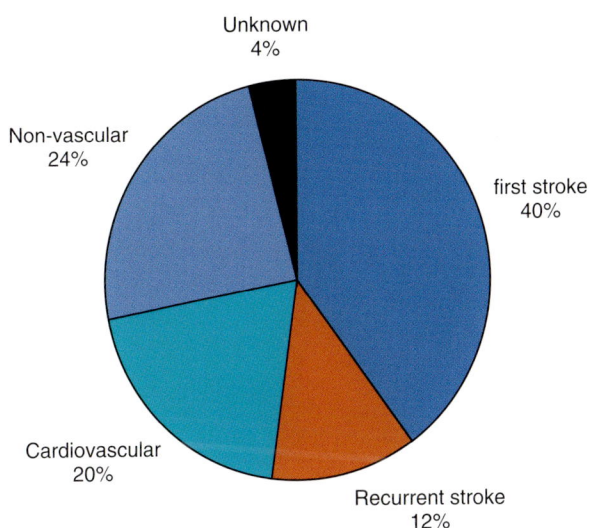

COLOR PLATE 2. Cause of death over 5 years following a cerebrovascular event. (From data of 370 patients of which 58% had died at 5 years, from Hankey GJ, Jamrozik K, Broadhurst RJ, et al. Five-year survival after first-ever stroke and related prognostic factors in the Perth Community Stroke Study. Stroke 2000;31(9):2080-2086). [*See* page 119].

Index

Printed in the United States of America